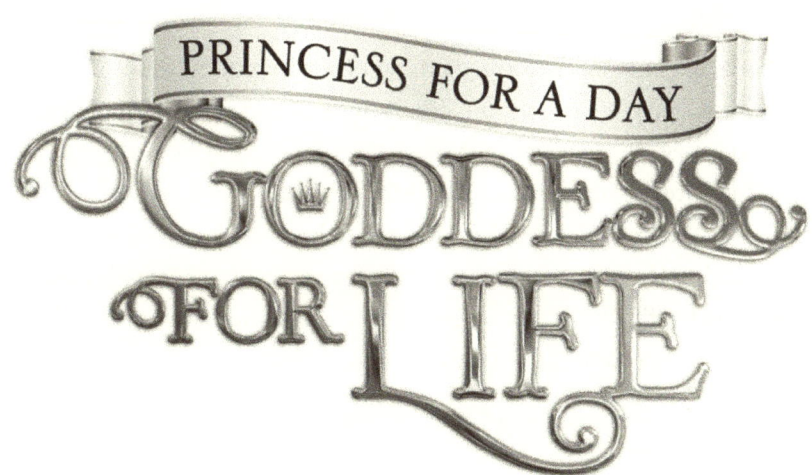

Princess For a Day, Goddess For Life
Shine On Your Wedding Day – and Forever After!

Anita Revel © 2012

ISBN 978-1-922165-04-6 (paperback edition)

All Rights Reserved, Anita Revel. AUSTRALIA

This book may not be reproduced in whole or in part by email forwarding, copying, fax, or any other mode of communication without author permission. The intent of the author is to offer guidance of a general nature to support your quest for physical, emotional and spiritual wellbeing. Neither the author nor the publisher will assume responsibility for actions you undertake for yourself or others based on information in this book. Please seek professional advice before making drastic decisions about your relationships.

Published by Now Age Publishing :: NowAgePublishing.com
PO Box 555, Cowaramup, Western Australia 6284

Cover by   Inspired Insight :: inspired-insight.com

Cover image   Sergey Galushko

National Library of Australia Cataloguing-in-Publication entry

Author:	Revel, Anita, 1968-
Title:	Princess for a day, goddess for life : shine on your wedding day, and forever after / Anita Revel.
ISBN:	9781922165046 (pbk.)
Subjects:	Brides.
	Self-actualization (Psychology) in women
	Self-realization in women.
	Women--Conduct of life.
	Weddings.
	Spiritual life.
	Happiness.

Dewey Number: 158.1

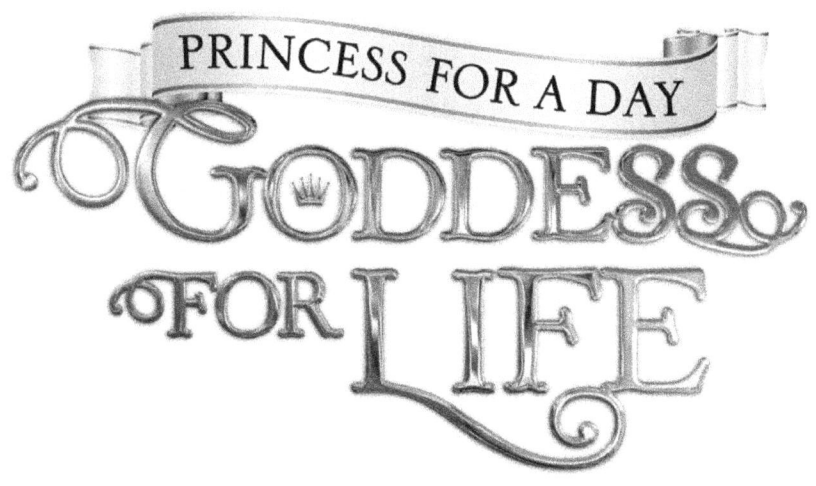

Shine On Your Wedding Day – And Forever After!

Anita Revel

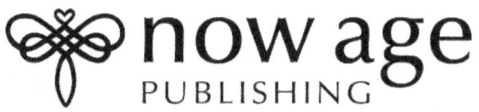

Table of Contents

Foreword   7

Princess For a Day   11

  The Way of the Happy Bride
    Beating the Post-Wedding Blues
  Attitude Rules
    Self-Centering Techniques
    Self-Appreciation Techniques
    Self-Motivation Techniques
  Body Rules
    Real Food
    Re-Hydration
    Rest
    Recreation

Goddess For Life   71

  Goddess Rules
    Be Present…
    Feel the Flow…
    Know Thy Self…
    Love Fearlessly…
    Speak the Truth…
    See Beauty…
    Understand Bliss…

In Summary…   95

Foreword

As a Civil Marriage Celebrant, I meet all kinds of brides. Relaxed ones, excited ones, calm ones, panicky ones, ones that believe in serendipity and ones that micro-manage every moment leading up to their big day. As unique as each bride is, however, there is one common trait they all share as it comes time to walk down that aisle – they are all acutely aware they are the centre of attention for the biggest, most important ceremony of their lives.

Every bride handles this attention and pressure differently. How she handles it is often a direct reflection of the type of lead-up she has had to her wedding.

Perhaps your life has been revolving around your wedding planning for the past 18 months. Or you've decided to elope and you've set the date for next month[1]. Regardless, as your big day gets closer and closer it's likely your stress levels and adrenalin will rise in proportion.

One purpose of this guide is to help you, the bride – the princess – "get it together" during the preparation and chaos

---

[1] Australian law requires that couples lodge their Notice Of Intended Marriage at least one calendar month prior to their ceremony and exchange of vows.

that seems to go hand in hand with planning such a big day, and more importantly, keep it together at crunch time.

But as we will discuss in further detail, there is more to getting married than having a blast on your wedding day. There's the post-wedding life to think about also…

This will arguably take more strength, persistence, patience and grace to pull off than the wedding itself. This is because there's no "big day" at the end with a huge party celebrating a turning point in your lives. There's just a daily, conscious commitment to stay in love with your spouse, to re-live your vows over and over again throughout the years, and the occasional bit of sacrifice to keep your boat afloat.

By all means embody the princess on your wedding day. It is every bride's right to do it her way. But read this guide in full before your day – it will show you how to remain connected with your inner goddess[2] during the process.

This will help you will achieve a healthy transition from single life to happy wife with poise and integrity intact. Doing so will help you slip seamlessly into the life of mutual support, healthy inter-dependence and deep trust with your soul mate for life.

If you're ready to step up and shine happily forever after, read on!

---

[2] An inner goddess, as defined in the *Inner Goddess Manifesto*, is "… a woman's guiding light, her sense of self, and her moral and behavioural compass. She's the force who enables the woman to enjoy life as a confident, capable, sacred and savvy human being"

*From today they shall call you
Co-travellers through life;
Adventurers and soul mates,
Husband and wife.*

"Declaration of Marriage"
~ by Anita Revel

Princess For a Day

Just say the word "princess" and it will conjure up various images and responses for different people.

There are the romantic princesses that dress in froth and bubble, are exquisitely beautiful, and get to marry their dream man (even if he was a frog to start with). They are sweet, angelic, see life through rose-coloured glasses, and generally need rescuing by a handsome prince – Disney's Cinderella, Sleeping Beauty and Snow White are examples of this type.

Then there are gutsy princesses who don't hesitate in kicking some butt and leading their kingdom with smarts – think Mulan or one of history's legendary queens, Queen Elizabeth.

Other princesses inspire compassion (Princess Diana); are natural champions of their people (Pocohontas); see beauty in everything (Belle / Beauty and the Beast); or desire normality above pomp and glamour (Jasmine).

And then there's the Princess Bride. In the 1987 film by the same name, Buttercup's farmhand responds to her every command with, "As you wish." We come to understand that the princess bride feels naturally entitled to have her wishes manifested by the man she loves. But that's not all…

The Princess Bride

The princess bride is every little girl's sparkly, magical dream come true. To be gazed upon with awe and love, to swan through the day feeling and looking beautiful, to be united with the prince of her heart in marriage forever after… A fairytale come true.

Whether she marries in a Church or barefoot on a beach, her dress is white or coloured, or she has many guests or none; the princess bride is the centre of attention during her ceremony and subsequent celebrations.

The gracious princess bride smiles from the moment she wakes because she knows, "Today I marry my love."

She has given thought to her vows because she knows they are for life. And she is the gracious host at the celebrations that follow because she is surrounded by the people she loves most in all the world.

Some brides take the princess factor to another level. Their focus tends to be on the wedding itself, rather than the marriage. This type is dubbed by the press as the *Bridezilla*.

The bridezilla embodies her vision of "Romantic Princess" right down to the last bauble on her tiara and sequin on her dress. She painstakingly coordinates her veil, shoes, jewellery, make-up, hair, spray tan, teeth-whitening and flowers… and not just for herself but also for her bridesmaids, flower girls, and sometimes her groom. Her wedding costs at least $50,000, even if it means going into debt or stepping on a few toes – as long as she gets the "perfect" wedding – her Big Day that she has been dreaming about since she was a little girl.

The Bride Who Cried

One thing missing from many brides' checklists and wedding plans, tends to be her post-wedding life. Planning her big day takes every ounce of her attention for countless months. Then, invariably she is overwhelmed with her status as "wife" not long after the last champagne bottle has been drained and the guests have gone home.

"What an anti-climax!" she cries. What will she focus on now? Where's the hype? What happened to her high-gloss Hollywood fantasy? Is she expected to live behind the white-picket fence now and behave like a Stepford Wife?

What happened to being a princess, where she was the centre of attention and everyone told her she was beautiful?

It's understandable that a princess bride thinks this way. After all, what do we see of Cinderella after she marries her Prince Charming? Or Ariel once she becomes Mrs Prince Eric? We are not privy to how they handle the daily chores that cause arguments ("It's your turn to do the dishes!"), challenges to their trust ("I swear, I didn't mean to stare at the waitress' butt!") or dilemmas that threaten their long-term security ("Sorry, I lost my job again.")

And so, dear reader, read on to keep your eye on the long-term plan… how to still feel like a princess even after the last party-popper has popped and your family has stopped calling you by your new family name as a novelty. This requires transitioning from a princess mindset, to a goddess one, and this guide will show you how.

Princess V Goddess

I once had a dream that I was in a reality TV show with Paris Hilton. The show was called *The Princess and the Goddess*. (Paris was the princess, and I was the goddess, in case you hadn't guessed already.) We were given different challenges to demonstrate how the different personalities handled them – like a princess on a pedestal, or like a goddess grounded in practicality.

I recall being more that a little jealous each time we landed at a different airport and Paris had an innate knack of rallying porter boys to collect her luggage and take it to a waiting limousine. Her princess nature just accepted that she would have people at her beck and call whenever she lifted her manicured finger. And while I was queuing at the hotel reception waiting my turn to check in, Paris was swanning past – her lackeys had already arranged to have her room key ready for her to head directly to her haven.

I recall wondering (in my dream) why was it that I couldn't command the same level of attention where people fell over themselves to make my way easy.

Perhaps, my dream Self told my perplexed Self, it's because being a princess only lasts for as long as the money, the fame and the notoriety is evident. Being a goddess, on the other hand, lasts for life.

Another analogy:

> *A princess is accustomed to being in the spotlight.*
> *A goddess **is** the spotlight, shining her light on the world.*

While Paris was getting all the attention, I was learning to be self-sufficient, considerate of others, generous with my kind words, and open to receiving back all the good vibes I was sending out.

I did this because being goddess means staying true to your core values, boundaries, self-respect and inner wow factor. Instead of the outer treats and trimmings that a princess' wealth buys her, a goddess is able to radiate a rich personality thanks to her inner wealth – she knows and accepts her Self on all levels; at a sub-conscious or DNA level she has confidence in her body, creativity and all-encompassing persona.

She is proud of her ability to love, communicate, trust, and understand her life lessons. She is balanced and calm in times of duress, playful and sassy in her approach to life, accepting of her shadow side when storm clouds gather, and a role model to younger women finding their way in the world.

In my dream, I knew that as long as I stayed resolute and aligned with my truth, that I would eventually win the challenges and ultimately, the Game.

And so it came to be I won this particular challenge… While Paris overspent her Game budget on room service and obligatory tips, I was given a complimentary upgrade to the penthouse. Turns out I'd made the concierge feel appreciated with a well-timed compliment – at the exact moment the penthouse became available. I knew there was a good reason I didn't have lackeys running ahead of me – it was just a matter of honouring my intuition to stay centred and connected with my inner goddess to find out why!

The Way of the Happy Bride

It is every girl's right to step into her princess role as much or as little as she desires. There is no doubt that on her wedding day, every bride looks incredibly beautiful, and is able to radiate her happiness with an effortless glow. But it's important to remember that all this work – all the organisation, manoeuvring, working out, detail management and stress – is for the sake of one day.

What happens after that day – once the princess glow has been washed off and the dress sent to the dry-cleaners – is dependant on how well you "come down" from the princess pedestal...

Being prepared to transition from princess to goddess will help you go from the stunning bride to lifelong wife with style – you'll be more balanced, better able to cope with change, and in a stronger position to negotiate with grace.

Let's start with getting prepared for the post-wedding day, with some strategies for beating the post-wedding blues.

Beating the Post-Wedding Blues

Ask any new wife what the biggest surprise about being married is, and one of her answers may allude to a feeling of anti-climax. "It was such a big day, it went by in a blur – all that planning for some hazy memories?!"

The following tips would have helped her make a healthy transition from single life to happy wife...

1. Focus on "Getting Married"

Do your invites read, "You're invited to our wedding," or "You're invited to celebrate our marriage"?

The nuance is subtle, but the difference is vast.

> *A **wedding** is the ceremony, usually followed by a reception or a celebration of some sort.*
>
> *A **marriage** is a commitment to another human being, to the exclusion of all others, voluntarily entered into for life.*

I am reminded of the bumper-sticker that says, "A puppy isn't just for Christmas." Despite being an adorable gift idea, the responsibility for the dog's wellbeing carries on far beyond the one day of celebration. In the same way, a wedding is for a day; marriage is for life.

It will help to remember that what you're planning for, is not a party-for-a-day, but a commitment for many more days, weeks, months and years!

2. Believe in Serendipity

One of my brides called me in tears the day before her wedding.

"Our accommodation was double-booked, and we've been packed off to an awful beach shack with nothing but a two-burner camp stove for a kitchen!" she sobbed.

The next morning she called to say, "Our florist has lost our order, and I woke up at 4am in a sopping wet bed thanks to my three year old son! Can my wedding day get any worse?"

Oh yes, it could… The ceremony started beautifully, with lovely personal words from the two witnesses present. Just before I was about to launch into the legal component, however, one of the witness' children declared her urgent need to go to the toilet. "Not just *ones*, daddy! *Twos!*"

The bride looked at me with a stunned expression, then burst into loud peals of laughter. "Why was I so fixed on having a *perfect* wedding day? *This* is perfect! I couldn't have scripted a better wedding if I tried!"

What happened to this bride was a release of expectations and a surrender to serendipity.

Serendipity is a pretty word describing a fortunate accident. At the time each thing that went wrong felt like a disaster, but in retrospect the bride was able to see the happiness that came out of each setback.

The beach shack meant she didn't have to worry about kids with sandy feet making the place dirty; the dismal kitchen facilities meant they went out for dinner and found their new favourite restaurant; the florist was so apologetic she gifted the flowers; the early-morning wake-up gave her extra time to walk on the beach and calm her nerves; and the child's announcement gave her the opportunity to laugh, release her stress, and reconnect with her groom through laughter. They ended up holding on to each other (more like holding each other up), and saying their vows through tears of joy.

3. Embrace the Transition

On your wedding day you are allowed to be a princess – in fact, most brides are expected to be one! The spotlight will be on you, the groom will defer many decisions to you, and you will look as beautiful as a magazine cover girl.

During your married life, on the other hand, the journey requires equal effort by you and your spouse. You will share the spotlight, (turning it to your children if/when they arrive), you will share the decision-making, and some days you'll have your hair in a scrunchie and sneak out of the house to do the school run in your tracksuit pants and slippers – a far cry from your big day as the princess!

Transitioning from Miss to Mrs can be dramatic – not in a bad way; just in a challenging way.

There may be a sense of grief at leaving your single life (and your "freedom" behind). You may feel utterly lost because you've never been in this situation before (the French call this feeling *jamais vu* – the opposite to *deja vu* – meaning, "never seen"). Also, after the adrenalin and climax of the wedding day, you may feel drained and broody, with the question, "What happens now?" on the tip of your tongue.

To transition gracefully, it's important to recognise the enormity of the transition required.

Take time to ease into your new role; and don't make any rash decisions until you're feeling completely settled – no new pets, no new real estate, and avoid cutting all your hair off! (Like I did!)

4. Take Time to Adjust

A honeymoon immediately after the celebration is vital for the healthy adjustment into a "married" frame of mind. Being alone together, enjoying each other's company in a stress-free environment, allows you to practice calling each other husband and wife; it lets you ease into a new relationship of lifelong inter-dependance; and it gives you time to explore your new "Self" as a Mrs – especially if you were worried that having a title of "wife" would usurp your personality. And, it gives you the space to come down from the adrenalin and hyper-happiness of the previous few months.

In the lead up to your wedding day, do give yourself time to imagine what it will be like to be a "Mrs". Thinking about it in advance will act like a shock absorber when you enter the transition – you won't feel so lost because you've already laid the foundations for familiarity.

When you become a wife, understand that it means much more than stepping into a 1950s housewife stereotype. Nowadays you can maintain your ambition and individuality; you can expect your spouse to share the workload, the housework and the decision-making; and, it will be up to you to gently guide and positively reinforce the dynamics of the family. You can do this best when you're happy – when you've worked out how to stay true to your values and honour your own needs.

Prepare to do what makes you happy (as long as it doesn't hurt your spouse or family), remembering that a "happy wife" means a "happy life" for all who live in your circle.

5. Keep Your Attitude Real

When movie star Jennifer Aniston revealed her engagement with Justin Theroux I was shocked at the "It's time she had some happiness" and "Now she's getting married she can be happy" style comments.

This is because marriage, in and of itself does not guarantee happiness.

Happiness in a relationship is about mutual respect, truth, guts and the knowledge that there is one person in the whole world who has your back. It's a deep knowing that you have a wingman for your awesomeness, a shoulder for your tears, and a balancer for your highs and lows. It's taking off the mask, baring your soul and opening your heart.

And, according to Nic Freeman, a Family Therapist (Free to be Relationships), it's about differentiation.

"Differentiation is the ability to know yourself and know what your needs are and be able to ask for those needs to be meet by a partner but also then be prepared to meet them yourself. Its about operating from a solid sense of self rather then a reflected sense of self where we look to the other to make us feel good about ourselves," she says.

"The Goddess Rules in particular are a practical guide for becoming differentiated, really getting to know yourself, so you can honour your needs and the needs of the other rather then look to the other to prop us up. This means we are more likely to be in a relationship for the right reasons, because of love rather then the ego of that person being there to make us feel good about ourselves."

Once you master the art of differentiation, respecting and loving the individuality of your soul mate *and* yourself, you can be confident you're entering marriage with a "keep it real" attitude.

You will be in a better position to understand that marriage can be a pitstop along the way, but it's not the pinnacle where you can say "Now we're married, we can be happy."

> *Marriage is a wonderful celebration of the journey so far, and a pledge to continue the journey forever.*

Only your inner sacred and savvy Self opened fully to the sacred and savvy soul mate and a willingness to forge ahead side by side, (or getting carried occasionally), will bring happiness in a relationship.

That, and buckets of self-respect, self-worth, self-fulfilment, and a willingness to support the same in your partner as he (or she!) supports you. These gifts do not come magically at the point of saying "I do." They are built over time, nurtured with trust, optimism and faith until they become part of the couple's DNA as a team.

I believe Jennifer and Justin have been working quietly, with dignity and determination, to build such a relationship, and they don't need a "marriage" for Jen to find her happiness. I believe she has had it within all along, and that Justin is the one who saw it, recognised it, and decided that this was the happiness he wanted to be a part of.

6. Keep The Sentiments Real

After three years of conducting wedding ceremonies I have noticed a trend in the types of readings and prayers couples are choosing to incorporate into their ceremonies. There has been a shift away from sugary, sentimental odes to love and marriage, and a tendency to choose readings that "keep it real" – readings that acknowledge that love isn't all plain sailing; there's the occasional storm to be weathered.

And so, based on my couples' preferences for ceremonies that are meaningful without being overly fluffy, here are my top recommendations for wedding blessings[3]

Oh The Places You'll Go: Dr Seuss

The opening stanza in this epic poem says it all:

> *Congratulations! Today is your day.*
> *You're off to Great Places! You're off and away!*

I absolutely adore this piece in a ceremony – especially watching moods lift and smiles broaden as everyone gets carried away on the wave of adventure and limitless life choices.

As it is long (around five minutes for the full version), it is best read by a friend accustomed to performance and theatrics, and who knows how to engage an audience with voice and gesture.

---

[3] Due to copyright laws I'm unable to reproduce the full text of prose that's not written by me, but you should be able to find the full versions simply by googling the prose title and author.

Fair Dinkum Love: Kim Cockerell

This poem was written by another Marriage Celebrant, located in Geelong, Victoria. Kim keeps it real in this catchy prose about what real love (as opposed to trophy love) is.

Fair dinkum love is not about romance or image or success.
Fair dinkum love is about two average people adoring
and accepting each other for who they are.

Hug O' War: Shel Silverstein

Couples with children (especially kids with a theatrical bent!) who want to involve them in the ceremony, choose this two-line ditty-style reading. It is easy for the kids to read, and never fails to get guests grinning.

The Art of Good Marriage: Wilfred Arlan Peterson

This is often read by the grandmothers or favourite aunties who have been married a while and can read this knowing it's the truth. The premise is that "happiness in marriage is not something that just happens," and, "It is not only marrying the right partner, it is being the right partner."

Weird Love: Dr Seuss

Not so much a reading as a quote, this appeals to couples with a quirky sense of humour.

We are all a little weird and life's a little weird, and when we
find someone whose weirdness is compatible with ours, we join
up with them and fall in mutual weirdness and call it love.

Right Now, Right Here: Anita Revel

This is a piece I wrote for my couples that has since been made into a song. (Check out Prita Grealy on iTunes.) It is my pleasure to include the full prose here – something I normally reserve as an "exclusive" for my couples.

Right now, right here; this moment is the culmination of a thousand moments – ordinary ones, magical ones, memorable ones, and perhaps ones that you'd rather forget!

Embrace them all, for it is the mix of all these moments that has made your relationship strong and deep enough to be here today.

Right now, right here; your relationship is entering a new phase. Who knew at the first glance it would lead to this moment of commitment? Deep down inside, I believe you both knew it!

Between that first moment and now, you have been co-travellers through life learning to trust each other, depend on one another, learn from each other, and love one another.

All of your experiences, your adventures, your dreams and your promises have been as individuals forging ahead, side-by-side.

But right now, right here; you will exchange promises that are a way of saying, "I still want to do all these things with you, but not as your boyfriend or girlfriend, or partner. I will do them as your husband; your wife."

Enjoy this moment Bride and Groom, for it is no doubt one of the magical ones you will want to keep forever!

Elemental Blessing by Anita Revel

This blessing is based on the Cherokee prayer, and was tailor-written for a couple who wanted to incorporate a subtle spiritual element into their ceremony.

At this time, here at this place and under this glorious sun, we are truly blessed by our mother earth, father sun, sister ocean and brother wind ... May these elements combined mean that you grow stronger together through the seasons, be always warm with the love in your hearts, never thirst for love or companionship, and sail through life safe in each other's arms.

Captain Corelli's Mandolin by Louis de Bernières

For the literature lovers, the paragraph that discusses the reality of love and passion is a popular choice.

Love is a temporary madness, it erupts like volcanoes and then subsides ... Love itself is what is left over when being in love has burned away, and this is both an art and a fortunate accident.

The Velveteen Rabbit by Margery Williams

A favourite childhood story for many, the discussion between Rabbit and Skin Horse strikes at the heart of what "real" is. Being real, can hurt sometimes, it doesn't happen all at once, and although *"by the time you are Real, most of your hair has been loved off, and your eyes drop out and you get loose in your joints and very shabby,"* it doesn't matter because the people that really love you only see your beauty.

Love by Roy Croft

Being part of a couple means respecting the individuality of the other, and appreciating that individuality for the qualities it brings out in yourself. Roy Croft sums this up with the opening line of his beautiful poem:

I love you,
Not only for what you are,
But for what I am
When I am with you.

Whatever Makes You Happy by Powderfinger

Couples often have a favourite song that is "theirs", that transports them to the place where they first met, the moment they first kissed, or the moment they first realised their hearts and souls were in true alignment.

Whichever song you choose to be read aloud in your ceremony, lyrics pack a punch when offered in the spoken word. This chorus by Powderfinger is a great example.

Dream on together, Leaning against each other
However it happens I hope, It's whatever makes you happy

7. Recall Your Commitment

There will be tough times during your marriage. Ask any married couple and you'll find that it's normal to have arguments. Many will add that "making up" is the best part!

These are simply a part of matrimonial growing pains. Don't stress them. Instead, re-visit the reason you fell in love in the first place. Recall the many shared moments that led you to the moment of commitment, and let each one of them touch your heart.

You may also plan ahead and incorporate a symbolic gesture into your wedding ceremony that will act as a "recall trigger" later on. This is something that will physically remind you, "Oh yes, this is why I married him/her."

Following are some examples of rituals that Marriage Celebrants are only too happy to include in their ceremonies.

Unity Candle / Coloured Sand

This ritual represents two lives (via the two separate candles) becoming one when the central "unity candle" is lit. The unity candle is displayed at home, and may be lit every anniversary with a mutual, private renewal of vows between the couple. Or, it may be lit during arguments to signal "Time out!"

There are various ways to incorporate a unity candle into a ceremony, but as many celebrants will tell you, only try this ritual indoors. For outdoor events it is recommended coloured sand be poured into one decorative bottle instead of using candles.

Love Letter in a Box

In the days leading up to their ceremony, the bride and groom each write a love letter to the other. During the ceremony they put their letters into a box with a bottle of wine (that's suitable for cellaring). The celebrant seals the box with instructions to open it again in one or five years time as a celebration on their anniversary and a way to revive the feelings they had for each other all those years before.

Truce Bell

A bell is blessed and the couple are instructed to keep it for times when there is discord in the home. If either the bride or groom feels it is appropriate to "call a truce" he or she will ring the bell. The couple agree that when this bell is rung they will take 10 minutes apart to "cool down" and return with a willingness to settle their differences.

Love Locks

Love lock, love-heart locks, wish locks, luck locks, or simply old-fashioned padlocks… whatever you call them, using a padlock in a marriage ceremony is symbolic gesture of everlasting love.

The story goes that once a couple close a padlock together, just as the lock cannot be unlocked, nor can their love and commitment to one another. If the padlock comes with a key, the key is tossed into a river (or ocean), or tied to a helium balloon and released during the wedding ceremony.

Visit yesidoweddings.com/with-this-love-lock-i-thee-wed/

8. *Prepare For Natural Cycles*

In his novel *Captain Corelli's Mandolin*, author Louis de Bernières describes love as "a temporary madness, it erupts like volcanoes and then subsides."

The Italians describe this thunderbolt of first love – this temporary madness – as *colpo di fulmine*, which translates to "stricken by lightening."

During this phase of a new relationship, energy is high, infatuation blinds, passion ignites and each moment is passed in the breathless anticipation of the next touch, the next word, the next smell, the next kiss.

Anybody who has been in a relationship more than a few years knows that this giddy stage does pass. If first love is the volcano eruption, then real love is what remains after the lava flow has passed. It is the transformed, nutrient-rich landscape upon which new foundations can be laid.

It may happen that during this second stage of a relationship a couple agree to commit to the other their lifelong devotion.

And thus comes the marriage. The Big Day. The turning point in their lives where the couple declare to the world, "This is the person with whom I shall share my sorrows, my joys, my dreams and my forever."

But "forever" is a long time! And within this forever there are more stages and cycles to come within the relationship. Here are some simple tips to prepare for each stage, and how to ride each one out.

Honeymoon Stage

You hold hands wherever you go, are not ashamed of PDA[4], still call each other sweety and darling, and you still get "that feeling" in your stomach when you hear their name.

Enjoy this phase, dear reader, but always bear in mind that all systems degrade over time without maintenance. (This concept comes from a law of thermodynamics, incidentally.) You must invest energy into developing a healthy maintenance system and begin habits that will help prepare you for the Three Year Glitch. It could be as simple as remembering to say, "Thank you," for the small things; "I love you," when you wake up each morning; and "How was your day?" when you arrive home in the evenings.

Yes, it can be as simple as that.

Three Year Glitch

In 2011, Warner Brothers conducted a survey of 2,000 adults in long-term relationships. The survey's purpose was to promote its film *Hall Pass*, but revealed cyclic clues that the honeymoon stage begins to fall flat after three years.

By this stage, you have lived with each other 24/7, pooled incomes or savings plans, had to schedule in romance to compete with busy lives, possibly had sleepless nights with a new baby, picked up countless toenail clippings from the rug, asked a thousand times to put a dirty dish in the dishwasher rather than the sink… And on and on it goes until the initial "thunderbolt" dissipates to a barely audible whimper.

---

4   Public Display of Affection

Research undertaken by the Pew Research Center[5] claims there are three significant factors cited by couples that keep their marriage alive. They are: faithfulness, happy sexual relationship and sharing the household chores.

What can be determined from this research therefore, is to stay loyal, stay sexy, and pitch in with the daily mondo!

Seven Year Itch

The term "seven year itch" was spawned by the 1955 movie of the same name starring Marilyn Monroe, and describes the inclination to stray after seven years of marriage.

Cyclically speaking, the human body renews itself over seven years in pace with the rhythm of our soul. This evolution is measured in physical steps – we have our adult teeth by the age of seven, we enter puberty at the age of fourteen, and adulthood at 21. By 28 our bodies look to become parents, and life epiphanies happen at around the ages of 35, 42, 49 and so on.

The same cycle of seven applies itself to relationships. What was new and exciting seven years ago (all-night partying on the beach) dies off and becomes a source of discontent (excessive alcohol and / or lack of sleep).

Fortunately, preparing yourself for the seven year itch will help you both sail through it. Plan a holiday or time out together to consciously re-connect, re-commit and re-call all the reasons you fell in love in the first place.

---

5   www.pewsocialtrends.org

9. *Follow the Attitude, Body & Goddess Rules*

When it comes to shining on your wedding day, then shining on for life, there are three sets of rules to get acquainted with: the Attitude Rules, Body Rules and Goddess Rules. In summary, they are as follows:

Attitude Rules

- ✓ Self-Centre
- ✓ Self-Appreciation
- ✓ Self-Motivation

Body Rules

- ✓ Real Food
- ✓ Re-hydration
- ✓ Rest
- ✓ Recreation

Goddess Rules

- ✓ Be Present
- ✓ Feel the Flow
- ✓ Know Thyself
- ✓ Love Fearlessly
- ✓ Speak Your Truth
- ✓ See Beauty
- ✓ Understand Bliss

Attitude Rules

The key to a healthy attitude is to remain centred in times of duress, align your attitude to self-appreciation, and draw on your authentic power within.

As such, this chapter examines tactics to bring yourself back to centre when the stress gauge rises. You'll also pick up some easy techniques to like the woman you see in the mirror, and get some ideas for motivating yourself to stay on track.

Getting Your Attitude in Gear

You probably know from experience how powerful your mind is and how it can affect your physical body. When we stress or become mentally fatigued, for example, our immune system reacts by weakening and making us more vulnerable to illnesses. Furthermore, we develop a lack of self-confidence which in turn results in low salary expectations, under-developed relationship skills (both personal and professional), and a feeling of "missing out" in all the good stuff other people seem to enjoy.

When you can see and tweak your attitude to a healthy one – one that lets you see the good in you and your world – you will find a new joy in treating your body like the sacred vessel it is. As well as finding a new natural glow that comes with self-respect, you'll feel more energetic and capable of taking on the challenges.

Self-Centering Techniques

Stress exacerbated by adrenaline, lack of sleep, PMS, caffeine overdose, all fuel your inner stress-head. You know the inner stress-head is stirring when your heart feels like it is burning or hurting, or there is churning in the pit of your stomach that makes you miserable. Sadly, she causes us to be brutal on ourselves and other people.

As women we feed that little inner stress-head far too much… Even you, in the lead-up to what should be the happiest day of your life, are probably stressing about work, about where money is coming from, making your relationship with your fiancée work, getting your head around being married for life, eating right, sleeping right, finding negatives in yourself about yourself, raising children if you have children, worrying about yesterday, worrying about tomorrow, and good Lord, the wedding!!! Oh yes, wedding planning really gets the gold medal for being a stress initiator. Craaaaaaaaaaaap!

The inner stress-head is roaring… and taking it out on your body – here comes the three dastardly **bl**ahs: the **bl**ack bags, the **bl**oating and the **bl**otchiness.

When you stress constantly, when you worry that nothing is going right, when you don't like yourself, you are causing your adrenals to go into overdrive, and then even in the calm, your brain can't make those hormones turn off.

Stress also shuts down your digestion, reproduction, and even your immune system to save energy. This is why stomach ulcers, skipped menstrual cycles, and your vulnerability to viruses and germs is so prevalent in those who stress so much.

Literally, by letting your inner stress-head get the upper hand, you are sabotaging your happiness.

The best way to tame this savage stress-head is to learn stress reduction techniques.

Following are a few simple tools and techniques for quietening the mind and turning down the inner critic.

In short, they are:

1. Meditation and yoga
2. Find your inner Pollyanna
3. Trust your intution
4. Become an affirmation goddess

1. Meditation and Yoga

Meditation and yoga are ways to connect with the divine and devote just a short period of time where your brain and body can take a break. They also decrease muscle tension, lower blood pressure and heart rate, increase alertness and let you connect with your inner divine.

Even if you can't set aside 30 minutes to meditate or do yoga each day, at the very least lay on a mat, arms outstretched, and melt into the floor. Lower your respiration and heart rate, and just be in the moment. Simply… *be*.

Breathing Meditation

Working with your breathing technique is one of the most effective (yet simple) ways that you can embrace the calm. It is your body's natural relaxation response.

The simplest way to "breathe" is to close your eyes and consciously breathe in deeply through your nostrils, then releasing your breath in a controlled manner out your mouth.

Keep breathing naturally through your nose. In, out, in out. Just breath normally, but acknowledge your breaths. Think about the actual feeling and sensation of the air going through you. This feeling is what your focus will remain on.

Monkey Mind Meditation

If you find that this makes your more fidgety and that your mind is more busy instead of less, don't worry, you are not doing mediation "wrong". You simply have what's known in meditation circles as a monkey mind.

One way around this is to simply acknowledge how busy your mind is, without judgement or self-criticism.

Try doing this for ten to fifteen minutes. You will find that your thoughts are subsiding. By the end of your session, you should find yourself more relaxed and energised. Your body has achieved a great sense of calm, and you won't be able to return to a busy mind again immediately.

Wide-Awake Meditation

This is an easy meditation style that doesn't require quiet space, or even a quiet mind. In fact, you have permission to have a busy head!

Instead of sending your attention inward (as with traditional meditation), Wide-Awake Meditation lets you send your focus outward. It allows you to become highly aware of everything happening around you, become appreciative of the people you meet every day, to see beauty, and to recognise your blessings.

If the world inside your head is noisy, cluttered or self-deprecating then you'll probably find the world around you is fractured and confusing. By realigning your focus to seeing a beautiful world, a beautiful world is what you'll manifest.

Moving Meditation

Yoga is primarily a combination of stretches, balance, and breathing, and this combination initiates your relaxation response. Find a great teacher who will support your efforts to reduce stress, and yoga won't be a luxury – it will be a *must*!

2. Find Your Inner Pollyanna

Pollyanna is 1960 Disney movie about a little orphan girl who is sent to live with her Aunt Polly after the death of her parents. Thanks to her father's encouragement to look for something to be glad about in every situation, (a practice she calls the "glad game") Pollyanna is an eternally optimistic and cheerful girl who becomes a cherished member of her new community.

Putting yourself in a "glad" mindset helps you see the positives instead of feeling glum about the negatives. Channelling your inner Pollyanna will help you see the bright side to an otherwise gloomy situation. Choosing positive and optimistic words will help the silver lining in the storm clouds will turn to gold!

3. Trust Your Intuition

This inner quiet voice of reason is your intuition – your gut instinct and innate sense of knowing. Intuition can be defined as your body's natural wisdom that knows what is right or wrong for you. When you can learn to trust your intuition, you can stop fretting over making decisions – your inborn wisdom is telling you exactly the right way to go.

The first step in trusting your intuition is learning how to hear or feel your intuition. For some people it is a voice, for others a sense, and for others a physical reaction. Sometimes it's all three at once. If you are new to listening out for your intuition, here is one very simple way to hear or sense it…

The technique? Tossing a coin. Yep, tuning in to your intuition can be that easy. Here is how to do it:

1. Think of a question that has only a **yes** or a **no** answer;
2. Hold the coin in your hand and assign **yes** to heads;
3. Toss the coin and check the result – is it heads or tails? (Therefore, is the answer to your question, yes or no?)

When you see your answer represented by either heads or tails, feel what your body is doing. Is your gut churning? Is your heart jumping with excitement? Is a voice wailing "Noooo!" or is it singing "Yes!"? Or perhaps you are itching to toss it again until you get a different answer? If you're feeling disappointed then you know the true answer to your question – the opposite to how the coin landed. But if your head is singing "Yes!" then you also know the true answer to your question – it is according to how the coin did land.

The truth is, the coin didn't give you your answer. *You* did. You simply used the coin as a tool for understanding your intuition, and from your intuition you got your decision.

4. Become an Affirmation Goddess

Thinking positive thoughts manifests in positive behaviour, attitude and outcomes. It also helps you be grateful for what you have, rather than being remorseful over what you do not.

Count your wins instead of your woes;
Count your blissings instead of your blows;
Count your friends instead of your foes;
Count yourself lucky to counteract sorrows.

Self-Appreciation Techniques

It is a hot topic that the media, fashion houses and society at large perpetuate the myth that a beautiful woman is thin, young and rich. Dove commissioned a study in 2005 and found that out of 3300 girls and women between the ages of 15 and 64 in 10 countries, 68 percent agreed that media and advertising set an unrealistic standard of beauty that they could not hope to achieve. It's important to remember that yes, models are beautiful, but again, they are only one kind of beautiful.

Thankfully the air-brush was unheard of when Rubens, Botticelli and Bouguereau were creating their fabulous works. They have inspired countless modern day works such as *Venice Reconstituted* by California artist Rip Cronk, or Baron Von Lind's stunning pin-ups, or the alluring burlesque performers that captivate audiences world-wide.

The rubenesque curves and ethereal goddess magnetism is one kind of beautiful. Slim and athletic is another. Tall and lanky is yet another, as is short and plump. No matter what kind of beauty you are, you will find elements of *your* divine by doing a few minutes of "Mirror Work" every morning.

Learning to like the woman you see in the mirror is a vital ingredient in the matrix of self-appreciation, self-acceptance and self-love. It beings with honing your attitude to one of acceptance. By way of illustration, let's begin with this little analogy, borrowed from my book, *The Goddess DIET, See a Goddess in the Mirror in 21 Days*.

The woman who stands in front of her mirror every morning and trash-talks her reflection, is the woman who goes to work and pigs out on the morning tea doughnuts.

"I'm fat and ugly anyway," she reminds herself. "Six doughnuts won't matter."

Oh, there might be a day when she denies herself any treats as a means of control. But deep down she knows that the more she resists the more she becomes obsessed with the sacrifice and the more likely she will gorge on it later. This woman's attitude is one of self-loathing, and keeps her in the "fat loop".

The woman who stands in front of the mirror and says nice things to her reflection, on the other hand, is pouring self-respect through every cell of her body. This self-respect filters through to her actions and choices throughout the day.

When the doughnuts are put in front of her, she takes only one. She enjoys her first bite because it is a treat, not trash. She may not even finish the doughnut, knowing that sometimes, one taste is enough.

This woman's attitude is one of self-appreciation. This is the essential ingredient to easy and permanent baggage-loss.

Here are two activities you can do to ditch the old habit of self-criticism and start seeing how beautiful you really are.

1. Beauty Is As Beauty Does

Look into a mirror first thing each morning. Hold your own gaze for a short period of time, and say meaningfully, "You are beautiful," or, "Hello goddess." Do not let any negative voice counter-act this statement. If you do hear the inner critic pipe up, repeat the exercise from the start until you feel a little flutter of agreement when you say / hear the words.

2. Acknowledge Your Beautiful Bits

Where your attention goes, energy flows. Focussing on a spare tyre only adds weight to the issue, (boom boom).

Express gratitude to your beautiful bits by affirming your reflection, and watch these 'bits' take precedence. Suddenly your round tummy is beautiful because you're looking at it with kind eyes.

When you lose attachment to 'ugliness', it loses it grip on you. Your body can then settle into its own perfect size, naturally and beautifully.

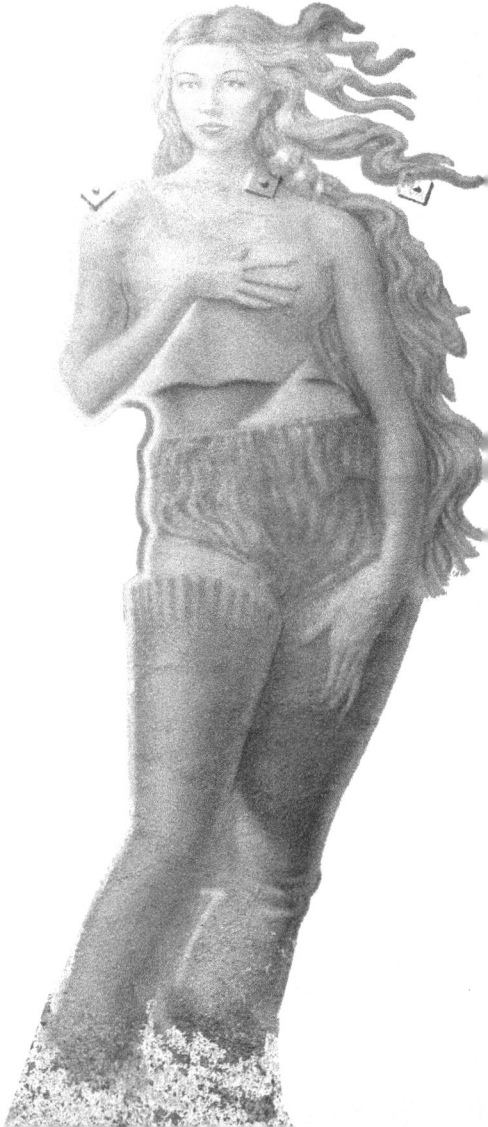

Image: *Venice Reconstituted* by Rip Cronk

Self-Motivation Techniques

Motivation is the desire to achieve a goal – in a bride's case it might be to lose (or gain!) five kilograms, to make her own dress, or to hand-write all the invitations. It comes to you in two ways: internal or external.

Internal motivation happens when you give yourself a pep talk, or find the strength within to keep going. Affirmations are a great tool for rallying inner motivation.

External motivation comes from outside influences, such as music, coaches, books and inspirational role models. You can consciously surround yourself with external motivation.

Without motivation to change weight, or to spend the hours on the dress-making or calligraphy, however, this bride is destined to turn up to her wedding with blotchy skin, a borrowed gown, and possibly no guests!

1. *Internal motivation: Affirmations*

An affirmation is a short, positive statement that describes an ideal outcome of a wish or desire. By identifying what you want from your life and expressing it in words as though it has already come to fruition, you are sending a clear message to the Universe of what you want it to provide.

The affirmation you choose must be a dedicated belief, not just an ad hoc approach to "trying it out". Choose an affirmation and work with it dozens of times daily in the lead-up to your wedding. Eventually you will find that because you've committed yourself to making this wish come true, your affirmation will come true.

There are many variations and outcomes possible. They can be spoken out aloud, recorded in your private diary repetitively, written on your computer screen saver, or written on individual sticky notes and hung around your daily environment.

Recommended Reading:

Affirmation Goddess – Express Your Way to Happiness (Now Age Publishing) by Anita Revel.

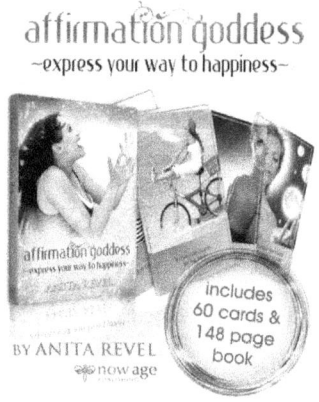

This collection of modern and sassy affirmations is founded on the seven states of wellbeing, with some additional "wild cards" to promote holistic wellbeing.

2. *External Motivation: Theme Songs*

Songs and music have long-been essential tools to help get athletes into a "winner" mindset. Athletes use music to block out internal noise; to help distract them from self-doubt and negative thoughts and instead reprogram their thoughts with positive, upbeat stuff. They often get into a "zone" before they compete using music to help them visualise what they are going to do during their performance.

American figure skater, Johnny Weir, listens to Edith Piaf's *Non, Je Ne Regrette Rien* (Regrets I Have None) before competing – there is something poetically beautiful about sweeping away the past, the pains and the pleasures, and "…

starting on new bases ... because my life, my happiness, today everything begins with you."

How appropriate for you as a bride, too, to have a theme song everyday of your workout to get you into a happy and positive mindset about your pending nuptials.

Or you could choose a song that simply makes you feel good whenever you need a pick-me-up. Use it as a crutch for every time you're feeling stressed or overwhelmed slip back into a good space by singing your theme song.

Here is a list of suggested theme songs to get you started[6]. Some will appeal to your inner goddess – that beautiful, sassy, soulful person you were born to be. Others are designed to get you dancing, helping you expel nervous energy. Yet others are simply there just to make you feel good!

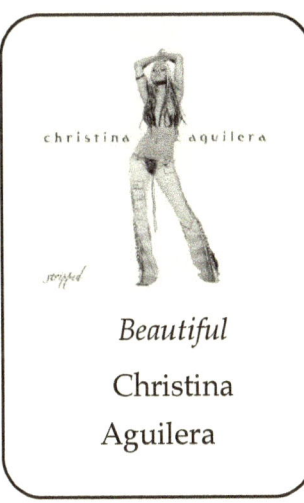

Beautiful

Christina Aguilera

"Cause you are beautiful; beautiful in every single way," sings Christina Aguilera. Every bride needs a personal uplifter for times when she is doubting herself, or having fears her dress won't fit, or perhaps because of a pre-marital tiff that has got her down. Christina reminds you that – girl, you are beautiful!

---

6   Search "theme songs for the bride to be" to read the full Listmania list at Amazon.com

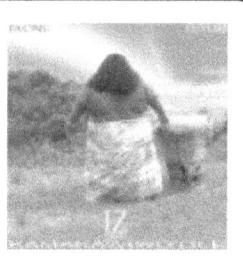

Over the Rainbow
Iz Kamakawiwo'ole

Israel Kamakawiwo'ole's version of *Over the Rainbow* features in movie soundtracks such as *Finding Forrester*, *Meet Joe Black* and *50 First Dates* for a reason – it is bright, uplifting and just makes a girl feel super happy! You'll be dreaming of Hawaii, blue skies and *love* before the song is even half-way through.

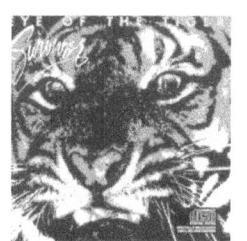

Eye of the Tiger
Survivor

I haven't met a bride yet who doesn't want to look toned in her wedding dress. This is the song that rocked Rocky Balboa through his punishing-yet-rewarding training regimes. Likewise it will help you push through yet another set of sit-ups, push-ups and epic stair-climbs. You can do it sister!

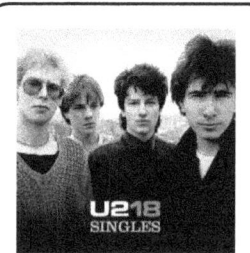

Beautiful Day
U2

For days when you wake up and the clouds are grey, the stress is building, the doubts are creeping in… This song by Irish super group U2, will help turn your focus from doom-and-gloom to a positive outlook. Suddenly, by focusing on a beautiful day, your day actually becomes one.

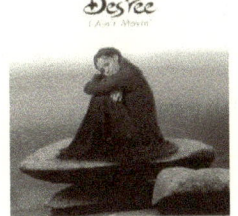

You Gotta Be

Des'ree

Got an interfering mother-in-law? Or a pushy wedding planner over-riding your decisions? Here's your theme song to give you courage… "… You gotta be cool, you gotta be calm, You gotta stay together…" and once you've regained your centre, well, "All I know, all I know, love will save the day."

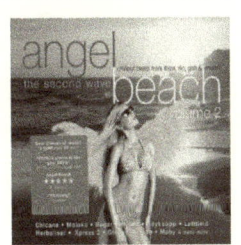

Breathe

Mulsanne

Every bride needs time out from the chaos surrounding her in the lead-up to the wedding. *Breathe* is the perfect track from the *Angel Beach* album to help you take five minutes and simply… *breathe*… Actually, the whole album is worth a listen, especially when five minutes of bliss just isn't enough.

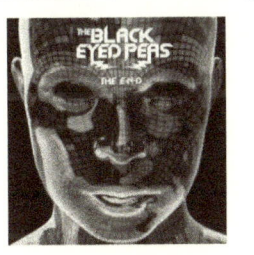

I Gotta Feeling

Black-Eyed Peas

The months of planning, the weeks of panic, the days of a thousand last details – the Big Day is here. Do you want your mood to be… "Has the salmon arrived, do the napkins match the plates, is Grandpa Grumpypants behaving…?" or do you want it to be "Tonight's gonna be a good, GOOD NIGHT!"?

Body Rules

There are four essential aspects of a healthy body, also known as the **Four Rs**:

1. Real Food,
2. Re-Hydration,
3. Rest and
4. Recreation.

1. **Real Food**

    Eat natural, unprocessed foods, and:
    - ✓ Eat slowly,
    - ✓ Complement and vary your foods,
    - ✓ Eat early, and
    - ✓ Detox and cleanse

2. **Re-Hydration**

    Drink up to two litres of water a day

3. **Rest**

    Get enough sleep, and take time during the day to relax, even if it for just five minutes. Incorporate play into your daily routine also. (Schedule time if necessary!)

4. **Recreation**

    Move that body sister! Whether it's structured sport or incidental fitness, see it as recreation / re-creation and have fun!

Real Food

Choosing real food is as simple as dividing food into two food groups – processed and unprocessed, or natural and unnatural. Make real food, rather than processed food or fast food, your priority for ongoing health.

Of course you will be tempted to eat on the fly as you run from appointment to appointment; you will be offered endless canapés and finger foods as you go from one pre-wedding party to the next; and you will probably find yourself reaching for the nearest snack food to throw down your throat in between phone calls.

Resist, resist, resist. Have fresh fruit in a bowl on the table. Cook up a large batch of vegetable soup and freeze individual portions for emergencies. Make rounds of sandwiches and freeze them – you'll be able to reach for them at a moment's notice when hunger pains hit.

If your goal is to develop a healthy glow from within, make wiser choices in your food selection. Draw your nutrients from a variety of sources, eat in moderation, and at the risk of sounding like a broken record, choose fresh, natural foods.

If you do slip and indulge in "Un-Real Food" there are two things you must do:

- ✓ Forgive yourself and move on;
- ✓ Increase your "Recreation" time. We will get in touch with the calorie tango in a moment, along with the most important rule: eat the goodness you want to feel.

Re-Hydration

Yes, you've heard it all before – you must drink around two litres of fresh water a day. Don't under-estimate the value of this advice – water is necessary to nourish your skin, organs, mind and attitude. It fills out your wrinkles (or 'laugh lines' as modern goddesses call them) and makes your skin glow.

The importance of hydration, and tips for how to drink eight glasses of water a day (without feeling bloated), is covered in my modern-day empowerment story for women: *BOTIBOTO: Beautiful On The Inside, Beautiful On The Outside – An Empowerment Story for Well-Rounded Women* (Now Age Publishing). Here are eight ridiculously easy ways to hydrate:

1. A glass upon rising;
2. A glass at breakfast;
3. A glass before leaving the house for work;
4. A glass upon arriving at work;
5. A glass at morning tea;
6. A glass at lunchtime;
7. A small bottle of water to sip at the red traffic lights on the way home, and
8. A glass before dinner.

I'm certain if you put your mind to it, you could find even more ways to include more water in your daily routine!

Rest

No matter how crazy-busy life gets, it's super important to grab 30 minutes of "Me Time" every day. Without it, you remain a slave to your routine, to others' demands and in the loop of stress.

The stress response, also known as the fight or flight response, is caused by an imbalance between your chaotic environment and how well you think you can handle it with what resources you have.

When you feel helpless, angry and directionless, these stress reactors cause your body to go into defence mode. Your adrenal glands kick in and release adrenaline and cortisol that give you bursts of energy to help you "flee" any perceived danger. When your body revs up those hormones it causes you to expend more energy than necessary for a very short time. As a result, your body reacts by immediately conserving energy and storing up fat by adding fats, sugar and insulin into your bloodstream. This cocktail makes it virtually impossible for you to lose weight.

Cortisol "…makes us store fat in case of famine," says David Cameron-Smith, Associate Professor in Nutrition Sciences at Deakin University in Melbourne.

So, stress = cortisol = fat storage. It also gives us a jelly belly as the fat gain tends to sit around the abdomen. The solution is to increase your exercise, recreation and Me Time to spark the release of beta-endorphins – brain chemicals which improve mood and promote calm.

Delegate! Tasks and Delegation Schedule

Decrease stress and increase "Rest" by delegating your jobs. Check which tasks you can delegate by ticking them off this list. Write next to each delegated task who you have delegated it to, and when you want them to have it done by.

Of course, you might not need every single bell-and-whistle on this list, in which case, white it out to make it look less intimidating! Remember, **Me Time** is more important than managing every task.

Apparel

- ☐ Gown _____
- ☐ Bridal shoes _____
- ☐ Bridal lingerie _____
- ☐ Hosiery / garter _____
- ☐ Jewellery _____
- ☐ Headpiece / veil _____
- ☐ Bridesmaid dresses _____
- ☐ Accessories _____
- ☐ Bridesmaid shoes _____
- ☐ Groom's tux _____
- ☐ Groomsmen tuxes _____
- ☐ Gown preservation _____
- ☐ Alterations _____
- ☐ Going-away outfit _____
- ☐ Honeymoon clothes _____
- ☐ Flower girl / Page boy _____

Flowers

- [ ] Bride's bouquet _____
- [ ] Bridesmaids' bouquets _____
- [ ] Corsages _____
- [ ] Boutonnière _____
- [ ] Reception centrepieces _____
- [ ] Altarpiece _____
- [ ] Pew/chair bows _____
- [ ] Flower girls' flowers _____
- [ ] Aisle chairs _____
- [ ] Rose petals for aisle _____

Stationary

- [ ] Invitations _____
- [ ] Announcements _____
- [ ] Map/direction cards _____
- [ ] RSVP cards _____
- [ ] Ceremony cards _____
- [ ] Save the date cards _____
- [ ] Postage _____
- [ ] Calligrapher _____
- [ ] Newspaper announcement _____
- [ ] Thank you notes _____
- [ ] Rehearsal dinner invites _____
- [ ] Hens invitations / event _____
- [ ] Bachelor party invitations / event ____

- ☐ Wedding programs _____
- ☐ Address labels_____
- ☐ Table diagram_____

Ceremony

- ☐ Officiant / Celebrant _____
- ☐ Personalised ceremony _____
- ☐ Original birth certificates _____
- ☐ Certified photocopies photo ID _____
- ☐ Location hire / permission _____
- ☐ Marriage license (NOIM[7])_____
- ☐ Wedding rings _____
- ☐ Altar decorations _____
- ☐ Certificate signing table _____
- ☐ Microphone, amplifier _____
- ☐ Chair/pew rental _____
- ☐ Pew/chair decorations _____
- ☐ Certificate signing pen_____
- ☐ Ring bearer pillow _____
- ☐ Flower girl basket _____
- ☐ Unity candle / sand vase_____
- ☐ Ushers _____
- ☐ Transport to service_____
- ☐ Transport from service_____

---

7 A "Notice Of Intended Marriage" is required in Australia. For step-by-step requirements for getting married in Australia, visit www.YesIDoWeddings.com

- ☐ Childcare_____
- ☐ Rice, petals, bubbles_____
- ☐ Insect repellent, umbrellas _____

Reception and Miscellaneous

- ☐ Location fee_____
- ☐ Caterer_____
- ☐ Food_____
- ☐ Musician_____
- ☐ Emcee_____
- ☐ Bar tender_____
- ☐ Liquor, mixers, H2O_____
- ☐ Security_____
- ☐ Guest book/pen _____
- ☐ Wedding cake _____
- ☐ Cake knife, servers_____
- ☐ Table decorations _____
- ☐ Other decorations _____
- ☐ Dishes, Glassware _____
- ☐ Napkins, Linens_____
- ☐ Tables, Chairs_____
- ☐ Parking_____
- ☐ Wedding favours_____
- ☐ Hair and make-up_____

Recreation

Australian national guidelines recommend 2.5 hours of moderate exercise a week – this works out to around 30 minutes a day. The United States Department of Agriculture recommends 60 minutes a day to prevent weight gain, and up to 90 minutes to help with weight loss. Here are some unique ways to exercise without the pain:

- ✓ See "recreation" as a chance for "re-creation" of your body, health and vitality.
- ✓ Adding just 2000 more steps to your day can prevent weight gain, says Dr James Hill at the University of Colorado Health Sciences Center. Walk your dog to the furthest tree for his wee, walk on the spot while watching TV, or pace while talking on the phone.
- ✓ Burn more fat by exercising in walk-jog-walk cycles of one minute each. You'll get a longer, easier workout than had you run flat-out from the start to the finish.
- ✓ Encore! Pretend you're the conductor of an orchestra. Their 'wing-flapping' motions give them an awesome cardiovascular workout.
- ✓ Dance! With his never-ending high-kicks, air-jumps, mid-air splits and energetic whoops into the mic, James Brown did the equivalent of a step class at every performance.

Certified Personal Trainer and Goddess Coach, Sandra O'Brien, has put together a Buff Bride pre-wedding workout program, as well as a Goddess-For-Life program that you can use for maintenance.

12-minute Workouts by Sandra O'Brien

> *You cannot outrun a pizza. You cannot out-train a bad diet. Eat to support your workout efforts*
> *~ Sandra O'Brien*

My name is Sandra O'Brien, owner and creator of the "muskoka goddess" system for women.

It is my goal that you find within yourself the ability to look and feel your absolute best, inside and out. I want you to feel powerful, unstoppable, able to effortlessly handle every curve life may throw at you. I want you to look at yourself and feel sexy and desirable.

My number one tip for your success is that you commit to working intensely at each and every workout. Never miss one.

This is your time to dedicate to looking and feeling your best in your dress. *Thinking* about it won't get you there; *doing* it will. So decide to do it, and commit to commit.

If looking hot on your honeymoon is important to you, you must do this. If you wish to walk down the aisle feeling like the most beautiful woman in the world, you must do this. If you want to breeze through your wedding preparations with less stress, you must do this.

Get it? You must do your workout every day. No excuses.

Each workout is only 12 minutes. Come on, everyone has twelve 12 in their day. You are important, the most important person in your life. No one can or will do it for you. There is no way around to achieving the body you want other than to just do it. You are worth 12 minutes – so take it!

Another tip is to make peace with the way your body now looks and feels. What "is" today, is nothing but a direct result of every action, meal and thought you have had up until right now. Accept it, love it, and know every day you are moving closer to becoming stronger, leaner and living a life full of vitality and joy.

How to gauge your intensity level – Scale 1 (at rest) to 10 ("I want to vomit")

For your safety, tune into your body and scale your comfort from one to 10. I do not suggest you push yourself to a 10. Listen to your body; it will always tell you how it is feeling if you are open to listening.

Every day your version of what, for example, a nine intensity level looks like will be different.

There can be many variables that affect your daily energy levels: the amount of sleep you had, how well you ate today or the past several days, hydration levels, time of the month, and so on. The important thing to remember is to always push yourself beyond your comfortable zone, without going to a 10 and feeling light headed and wanting to vomit.

Don't allow your mind to talk you out of working to the very best of your ability during each and every workout. On the days where you just don't feel like working out, commit to doing it anyways. Doing something is always better then blowing it off completely. Each and every workout you do adds up to you creating your sexy, lean, yummy body and having you that much closer to walking down the aisle and feeling like the Goddess you are. And, of course, feeling extra desirable on your honeymoon – *the* most important part of your wedding experience… I'm just say'n'!

Time to Workout

You have two main workouts that you are to complete over a seven day period.

Workout 1 is to be done on Monday, Wednesday and Friday. **Workout 2** is to be completed on Tuesday, Thursday and Saturday. Sunday, you are to complete the butt and abs routine.

You are also to complete the butt and ab routine at least two other times during the week. You can do this right after your main workout for the day or at another time of the day that works with your schedule.

How many weeks will be required before you achieve your ideal body, will depend on how far you currently are away from your goal.

Many factors will contribute to your success – how cleanly you eat, how intense you workout, your consistency and commitment to completing daily workouts and your mindset.

I have written a detailed description of each exercise in the following pages. You can also see each exercise, (and the cool down), demonstrated on my website muskokagoddess.com.

If you require further clarification of movements, please feel free to email me directly via muskokagoddess.com

Warm Up

Complete a warm up before every workout. You'll find a practical demonstration via muskokagoddess.com.

- ✓ 20 jacks
- ✓ 3 full body circles each direction
- ✓ Side to side twists
- ✓ 3 soldier swings, 3 diagonial swings, 3 hugs across body
- ✓ 3 front back leg swings, 3 diagonal swings each side
- ✓ 3 hip rotations forward, 3 reverse, each side
- ✓ 10 squats
- ✓ 3 down dog , up dog
- ✓ 10 side to side lunge
- ✓ 3 burpees

Buff Bride Workout #1

Monday, Wednesday, Friday

1. Burpees 10

From a standing position jump up, crouch down so hands are on the floor in front of you, drive your legs behind you so you end up in intermediate plank position. Shoulders square, chest is lifted, belly button is pulled in and up towards your rib cage. As you exhale, bring your knees back to your chest into a crouched position and explode up into an upright position. Jump to the sky at the top of the movement and repeat.

2. Jump squat 10

Feet are hip width apart. Lead with your glutes/butt as you lower your hips toward the floor. Ideally your quads are parallel with the floor. Weight is on your heels, chest and eyes are forward. Push through your heels and jump as high as you can, heels leave the floor. Land softly, toe, heel. Bend your knees as you land to absorb the shock. Inhale down and exhale as you jump.

3. Push ups 10

From an intermediate plank position, hands are shoulder width apart or slightly wider, elbows are straight. Lift your chest, pull your shoulder blades down. Legs are strong and straight. Toes are tucked under. Engage your core.

Lower your chest towards the ground so your biceps are parallel with the ground. Exhale and push back to start. For beginners, I suggest lifting from your knees.

4. Hip raises with alternating knee squeeze   10

Lay on your back with knees bent, feet flat on the floor. Push your hips toward the sky, pushing through your heels and squeezing your glutes at the top. Inhale and lower your glutes to just above the ground. On the next hip rise, bring your knees together as you squeeze your glutes. Lower the movement and push through the heel again, squeezing your glutes at the top. Lower your hips and squeeze knees together at the top of movement again. Bring knees together on alternative raises. Inhale down, exhale up.

5. Repeat

Complete as many rounds with fabulous form as you can in 12 minutes. Work intensely, rest when you need to and get back at it for the remainder of the 12 minutes.

Get comfortable in your 'uncomfortable zone". Pushing yourself is where the changes will occur in your body. Breathing hard, making noises, grunting, groaning and yes, even swearing (if you are so inclined) is where you need to be to make lasting changes in your body.

Buff Bride Workout #2

Tuesday, Thursday, Saturday

1. Back lunge with front kick, alternating   20

From a standing position, bring your left leg behind you as you bend your front leg, front quad parallel to the ground. Weight remains mostly on the heel of the front leg. As you push off the heel of the front leg, drive your right leg forward into a kick, pushing through the heel. Think more Bruce Lee, not Can Can. Keep your shoulders stacked over your hips as you kick.

2. Superwoman with hands behind head   10

Lay face down on the ground, hands behind your head. Lift from your hip flexors to lift your legs off the ground. At the same time lift your chest off the ground. Squeeze your shoulder blades back as you rise, head remains in line with your shoulders.

3. Side lunge with hop   10 per leg

From a standing position, step your left leg to the side of your body and place on the ground so your shoulder, hip, knee and ankle are in alignment. Push through your left heel and bring your knee up towards your chest, back to starting position. Step the leg out again in correct alignment and repeat. Keep your spine long and chest up throughout the movement.

4. Suicide plank   10

Lie face down on the ground. Tuck your toes under and balance your weight on your straight arms, so you are in intermediate plank. Ensure your hands are directly under your shoulders. Pull your belly button up towards your rib cage to support your lower back. Drop your left elbow to the ground then your right so you are in plank position. Push back up to intermediate plank with your right arm, then left. Drop to the ground again, left, right. Repeat, keeping your hips are square as you can.

Legs, hips, butt and stomach Workouts

Sunday + two other days

Bonus Workout #1 should take around 12 minutes. Complete as many rounds as possible in the allotted time

- ✓ Dogs, 16 per side left and right
- ✓ Bikes, 16 (left right is one count)
- ✓ Up and Over, 16 per side left and right
- ✓ Bikes, 16 (left right is one count)
- ✓ Straight leg pulses to shoulder, 16 per side
- ✓ Straight leg circles, 16 per side to be done immediately after the toe to shoulder movement above
- ✓ Bikes, 16 (left right is one count)
- ✓ Bent leg – Glute Raises, 16, immediately followed by
- ✓ Straight leg foot to butt, 16 per side
- ✓ Bikes, 16 (left right is one count)

Bonus Workout #2 is also 12 minutes. Again, complete as many rounds as possible in the allotted time.

- ✓ Sumo squat, 16
- ✓ Cross mountain climbers, 16
- ✓ Side lunge with hop, 16 left and right
- ✓ Cross mountain climbers, 16
- ✓ Back lunge with front kick, 16 left and right
- ✓ Bugs, 32

Goddess-For-Life Workout

Congratulations! You've got hyped, hot and healthy in time for your wedding day. That's no excuse to quit working your body, however. Oh no no no – keeping fit is a life-long pursuit.

It doesn't have to be difficult though. That's why I've come up with a simple routine that you can fit into every day as easy as pie. It's called the Goddess-For-Life Workout.

Again, I've recorded this workout so you have a visual guide as to what to do. You can view the video via muskokagoddess.com

The Workout

- ✓ Jumping jacks: beginner 20, advanced 100
- ✓ Full body wave with squat, 10
- ✓ Full body circles, 3 each direction
- ✓ Large hip circle/small hip circles, 4 each direction
- ✓ Downdog to updog reps: beginner 5, advanced 20
- ✓ Reverse table top up/down: beginner 5, advanced 20

- ✓ Plank with knee drop, 20 left-right equals 2 counts
- ✓ Side lunge with hop: beginner 5, advanced 20. Complete all reps with right leg, then complete with left leg
- ✓ Quad burn: beginner 10, advanced 30
- ✓ Ham burn, single leg / both legs: beginner 10, advanced 30. If this is too difficult, you may keep both feet on the ground for a hip thrust until you are stronger and able to do the single leg ham burner.
- ✓ Cross mountain climbers: beginner 10, advanced 50
- ✓ Bicycles: beginner 16, advanced 50+

Cool Down

Roll onto all fours, tuck your toes under and push back in to down dog. Push your tail bone up to the sky, lengthen your spine and keep your ears between your biceps. Bend your knees and walk your hands back towards your feet. Grab opposite elbows and hang like a rag doll. Shake your head out yes and no. Weight is on your heels. Put as much bend in your knees as you need. This should feel good!

Ensure your feet are a little wider than hip width apart, weight on your heels. Pull your upper body over to your right leg. Think of folding in half, lengthening your spine, belly button to top of leg versus chest to knee. Reach the crown of your head as close to the ground as possible. Lift your right arm up towards the sky, eyes follow your fingers. Open up your chest and squeeze your shoulder blades together. Breathe. Hold for three breaths. Repeat on the left leg.

Walk your hands out to down dog, feel an extra stretch in the back of your legs. Lift your left leg to the sky, flex your heel back, drop your foot back towards your butt. Stack your hips on top of each other and look under your arm pit. Lift your knee high and breathe. Swing your left leg through to pigeon pose. See diagram to the right. Keep your back leg straight and engaged, femur facing the ground and lengthen your leg, attempting to get your foot as far away from your hip as possible. Fold your body forward over your left leg. Relax your head and shoulders and breathe. Hold for five breaths. Take your left arm and place it under your right, shoulder on the inside of your left thigh.

Tuck your toe under and push back in to down dog, repeat on the right leg. Bend your knees so you are on all fours on the ground. Move your hips back towards your heels and relax in child's pose.

Spend a minute or two in child's pose to breathe and thank your body for supporting you in all you do every day. Thank it for being strong, healthy and beautiful.

Roll on to your right side, and push yourself up to a seated position. Close your eyes and just be. Settle and listen to your body as it breathes, with no effort from you.

Inhale slowly to a count of five. Fill your lungs with life giving breath, and hold for a slow count of five. Open your mouth and exhale for another count of five.

Pull your belly button back towards your spine and exhale every last amount of air from your body.

Goddess For Life

Now that you've aligned your attitude and acquired some healthy body guidelines, it's time to turn our eye to the bigger picture. What happens after the wedding day? How do you go from single woman to lifelong wife? How to retain your beautiful personality, individuality and glow – for life?

The answer is to discover, connect and honour your goddess within – the beautiful, sassy, intuitive, loveable, sacred and authentic Self that we were born to be.

According to the Inner Goddess Manifesto[8], "A woman who knows and accepts herself on all levels is fully connected to her Inner Goddess."

The term denotes the feminine aspect of a woman's psyche. This aspect is unique to women – not just in our body shape, function and our "bits", but in the way we love and nurture others *and* our Selves.

We were born to love and respect ourselves but many of us were conditioned to be humble, effectively becoming slaves to the inner critic. How wonderful would it be that in loving ourselves – our gifts, quirks, weaknesses, strengths, ambitions,

---

8   The *Inner Goddess Manifesto* is available as a free download from iGoddess.com

creativity and sense of humour – we inspire others rather than making them jealous or judgemental?

In loving the inner goddess, we are allowed to be as vulnerable and soft, or strong and brave, as we are inclined to be. No-one judges us for our choices, because in being true to ourselves we inspire others with our honesty and light.

Reconnecting with the inner goddess gives us permission to receive as much love as we give and deserve. In being free to love unconditionally – both ourselves and others – we are allowing our inner goddess to flourish.

Women have different ways of thinking, feeling, processing and dealing with situations. We also have physical differences that affect the way we act, what we do for a living, how we nurture, and what motivates us to move.

When a woman is able to transcend inhibitive social expectations or perceived behavioural requirements and instead act in a way that is fulfilling for her, she is honouring her inner goddess.

The inner goddess is a woman's guiding light, her sense of self, and her moral and behavioural compass. She's the force who enables the woman to enjoy life as a confident, capable, sacred and savvy human being…

How does a woman reconnect with her inner goddess? One easy way is to acquaint yourself with the seven basic Goddess Rules, and adopt them as your "rules of engagement" in everyday life.

Goddess Rules

A woman who knows and accepts herself on all levels is fully connected to her Inner Goddess. There are seven levels of self-awareness, knowledge and behaviour:

1. **Be Present**

    Celebrate your physical body and your connection to Earth, family and humanity.

2. **Feel the flow**

    Become comfortable with infinite abundance, emotional flow and creative freedom.

3. **Know Thyself**

    Be proud of your Self and your actions in all aspects.

4. **Love Fearlessly**

    Foster mutually fulfilling relationships at all levels.

5. **Speak Your Truth**

    Be heard by speaking with authenticity and diplomacy, and share your learnings with grace.

6. **See Beauty**

    Clearly know what is right for you, and act in honour of your innate wisdom and intuition.

7. **Understand Bliss**

    Open yourself to joy; revel in your divine purpose/ work with gratitude, dignity and generosity.

Be Present…

One of my brides confided in me that in the lead-up to her wedding day, she felt caught up in everyone else's dramas. In particular, her bridesmaids were in-fighting and jockeying for "top dog" position in the line-up. Her mother was dropping endless hints to invite their own friends to the reception (to the point of coercion). And, she felt as though her fiancé was running to a different agenda with his night-after-night of parties and poker nights. She felt isolated, began losing sleep, and reached the point of wanting to run away.

"If you're feeling flighty and disconnected, it's time to get grounded," I gently advised. (I don't like giving advice, generally, but this bride was practically strapping on her running shoes!) "This means getting back into your body and in touch with who you really are and what you really want."

When you are grounded, you are "present". You can:

- ✓ Celebrate your physical body because you feel settled, centred and that "all is right in your world" ;
- ✓ Eat well, be well, and feel comfortable in your skin;
- ✓ Forge ahead because deep down you know you're on the right path;
- ✓ Carve your own path and lead by example;
- ✓ Respond to threats and chaos with rationality and calm;
- ✓ Be more connected with Mother Earth and humanity;
- ✓ Consider yourself a valuable member of your community;
- ✓ Uphold the traditions of your tribe – your ancestors, friends, community and of course, your new in-laws!

Ways to be more present...

- ✓ Stand barefoot on natural ground. Feel the texture of the earth, grass or sand under your feet. Give thanks to Mama Earth for sustaining you in a state of security and health.
- ✓ Sit under a tree and imagine your spine extending downwards, into the earth, meshing with the roots of the tree and establishing you as an essential part of the eco system. Meditate upon feeling well, happy and grounded.
- ✓ Research your family tree and portray it in a line-drawing, collage, painting, patchwork quilt or any other creative manner. Reflect on your valuable role within this matrix.
- ✓ Physical activities include stomping, walking, hiking, standing in a warrior pose, and dancing.
- ✓ Create an affirmation and repeat it often. Key words can revolve around feeling safe. Themes for release include insecurity, invisibility, boredom, disconnection or impatience. Take on a goddess role model that represents the "Warrior Queen" archetype. Being earth goddess is about being in tune with your physical body, and being able to respond to threatening situations rationally and calmly. It also means giving back to Mother Earth her nurturing in equal measure. Role models include Kali, Freja, Cordelia, Gaia, Lilith, Artemis, Venus.
- ✓ Use essential oils to bring you back to centre. The Goddess-ence 100% pure essential oil blend for the base chakra uses ginger to boost self-confidence, lavender, patchouli and palmarosa for their calming properties, and grapefruit white to energise and uplift willpower.

Feel the Flow…

The flighty bride set out to purposefully and willingly get grounded. First of all, she sat and meditated under a tree. She turned off her phone, breathed deeply, let her mouth curve upwards slightly, and began.

Under this tree, she visualised herself walking down the aisle, being surrounded by the smiling faces of her nearest and dearest, and stepping easily forward to the side of her groom. On this trip down the imaginary aisle, she noticed something: she could only see the face of the one person in all the world she loved the best. The bridesmaids, the mother, the mother's friends – none of them took priority in her consciousness. They simply melted away as her groom's face came more and more into focus.

With every step her body relaxed more, and she remembered what this day was all about. It didn't matter what her bridesmaids or mother did to pressure her. It didn't matter that her fiancée was enjoying his mates' company. (She respected his free will, after all.)

Her day was about getting married; not putting on a show!

Checking into her gut feeling – her intuition – she knew this was the right path for her. In the act of intentionally becoming more grounded and more present, she was able to see the bugbears for what they really were: distractions.

This in turn empowered her to take charge of her own destiny once again. As if by magic, the bridesmaids tuned in to her new-found power and fell into line without a whimper.

As for the issue of her mother wanting to invite family friends, however, my bride still felt uneasy.

"Why don't you just go with the flow and see what happens?" I suggested.

When you can step into the flow of the Universe you can become comfortable with infinite abundance, emotional flow and creative freedom. You can:

- ✓ Accept and manage change gracefully;
- ✓ More easily release any need to control external forces;
- ✓ "Go with the flow" in line with your purpose;
- ✓ Attract abundance which is exactly right for you;
- ✓ Relish beauty, embody grace and attract both attributes;
- ✓ Nourish yourself with enough sleep, good food, fresh air and time for your passions and hobbies;
- ✓ Release attachment to expectations, open yourself to all possibilities, allow emotions to run their course, and ignite the divine spark that resides within.

So, my bride made "FLOW" her mantra for the week. Nothing would trouble her, upset her, or cause her to get sucked back into the distractions of planning a wedding. That was her promise to herself.

Thereafter, in answering her mother's pleas to invite extra friends, she simply replied "Whatever!" in a breezy, happy-go-lucky way. Lo and behold, she suddenly didn't care any more. It wasn't going to make or break her happiness if extra people were there. Only she and her groom could be responsible for their happiness. Problem solved, and everyone moved on!

Ways to feel the flow...

✓ Do something playful – squeal your way down a slide, swing a hula hoop around your hips, go body-boarding in the surf, play hopscotch, scribble and doodle a full page in your journal.

✓ Prepare a scrumptious, nutritious meal. Bless your food before eating, and give gratitude with every mouthful for the many miracles that brought this food to your plate.

✓ Take a belly-dance or zumba class; don't give a toss about how funny you might look. Other physical activities include shimmying, playing, eating, de-toxing.

✓ Key words for an affirmation can revolve around fun, play, sexuality, joy, femininity, freedom, flow, trust, permission, abundance, prosperity and creativity. Themes for release include control, fear, prudishness, self-loathing, self-judgement, creative block and depression.

✓ Take on a goddess role model that represents the "Magical Muse" archetype and the domains of self gratification, creativity, abundance and the feminine divine. Goddesses such **as** Ishtar, Baubo, Ceres, Tyche, Aphrodite, Ostara and Sri Laxmi show us how to creatively, emotionally and sexually, connect with others through feeling, desire, sensation and movement.

✓ Use essential oils to raise your self-appreciation vibes. The Goddess-ence 100% pure essential oil for the sacral chakra uses ylang ylang for its anti-depressant qualities. Sweet orange and grapefruit white relieves anxiety and patchouli is used for its calming effect.

Know Thy Self...

Earlier I mentioned the concept of differentiation. It's that quality in a relationship that means getting to know yourself fully so you don't look to your partner to complete you.

One implication of this is retaining your individuality and all the values and qualities that made "you" the person your fiancée fell in love with in the first place. It also means respecting, encouraging and loving the individuality of your partner, but for now, we are focusing on *you*.

When you know who you truly are, you can be proud of your Self and your actions in all your aspects. You can:

- ✓ Live, breathe and present your authentic Self to the world;
- ✓ Be absolutely real in whatever role you take on in life;
- ✓ Allow your inner wisdom (or intuition) to guide your decision-making and actions;
- ✓ Be intrinsically connected to your intuitive Self;
- ✓ Set clear boundaries and have them respected;
- ✓ Know that anxiety and 'butterflies' that sit in your belly is simply your inner tigress preparing you for success;
- ✓ Understand you are responsible for your own actions and your reactions to others.

It's like Shakespeare said. "To thine own Self be true." At all times, check in to your intuition – your in-built guidance system – and honour it. Set boundaries and be ready to defend them. Be proud of who you are and the qualities that you bring to your relationship. Following this advice will make you more (em)powerful than you could ever have imagined.

Ways to know yourself better...

- ✓ Surround yourself with yellow to improve digestion and appetite, and to bring some sunshine on cloudy days.
- ✓ Grow sunflowers and dandelions to remind you of your youth, joy, sunny nature, and resilient strength.
- ✓ Stress is often harboured in the solar plexus chakra – you may get a knot in your stomach, or you can have a 'gut-full' of a situation. Certain foods such as complex carbohydrates help regenerate the feel-good hormone, serotonin, which otherwise drops during periods of stress.
- ✓ Physical activities include hula hooping, intuition development, roaring like a tiger, abdominal exercises.
- ✓ Affirmations revolve around reclaiming power, keeping power and being empowered. Also look at integrity, authenticity, respect and self-worth. Themes for release include manipulation, anxiety, fear and self-loathing.
- ✓ Take on a goddess role model that represents the "Daring Diva" archetype. These goddesses show you how to delve deeper than the superficial exterior: Pele, Astarte, Oya, Diana, Bodicea, Maia and Persephone, and encourage you to be responsible for your own actions.
- ✓ Use essential oils to make you more alert and in sync with your body. The Goddess-ence 100% pure essential oil blend for the solar plexus chakra uses lemongrass and eucalyptus cleanse and decongest, rosewood for its restorative qualities, peppermint for stimulation, bergamot to uplift, and lime and lemon myrtle to promote clarity and assertiveness.

Love Fearlessly...

It is in human nature to flourish in the company of others. If we're lucky, out of all the human beings in all the world, we get to find that one person – the "soul mate" – who strikes the chord in our heart that renders it loyal to that one person only.

George Eliot (the pseudonym of Mary Anne Evans), describes this connection between two people beautifully.

> *What greater thing is there for two human souls than to feel that they are joined for life, to strengthen each other in all labour, to rest on each other in sorrow, to minister to each other in all pain, to be with each other in silent unspeakable memories at the moment of the last parting?*

Indeed, humans are built for companionship. But how to find that person – the lifelong companion – in the first place? The confidante with whom physical and emotional intimacy is a joy; the life-long friend with whom play and adventure come easily; the trusted partner with whom it is a pleasure to raise a family?

And what if you've found your one-and-only already? How to maintain your individuality within your relationship? To retain your essence, keep your love alive, and foster a healthy balance between dependence, inter-dependence and independence?

I like to think that the answer lies within your ability to love fearlessly, not only outwardly, but inwardly also.

When you are loving fearlessly you can foster mutually fulfilling relationships at all levels. You can:

- ✓ Embody love, compassion, grace, gratitude and trust;
- ✓ Happily share these qualities with others and receive them back unto yourself;
- ✓ Enjoy first-class treatment by others, because second-best isn't in your vocabulary;
- ✓ Attract respect naturally when you behave with self-respect, self-love and self-appreciation;
- ✓ Be the go-to girl for friends, in good times and bad;
- ✓ Break down walls made of fear, guilt and mistrust;
- ✓ Raise well-adjusted children with healthy self-esteem;
- ✓ Invite in joy, reciprocated love and trust at a deep level.

Signs that your level of self-love is flagging include looking in the mirror and criticising perceived imperfections, refusing to accept compliments, and flying under the radar because you fear you're not "good enough".

Make a note of any self-bashing behaviour this week: when you experience regrets, fears, guilt, self-loathing or distrust.

For example, you might berate yourself for napping when you have 100 invitations to write. Or you feel guilty for giving your wedding planned another job to do, or you regret not speaking up about an issue that's important to you.

Consciously strive to turn these words and actions around. Congratulate yourself for taking a nap when needed; for using diplomacy with the wedding planner; and for resolving to address the issue that needs your attention.

Ways to love fearlessly...

✓ Give yourself a pat on the back for being the beautiful, sacred and savvy human being you were put on this earth to be. Sticky-tape this message to your mirror (or somewhere you'll see it often) so you don't forget!

✓ Watch videos that make you cry! (With happiness, that is!) Here are some of my favourites on YouTube (http://www.youtube.com/playlist?list=PLA127DF6F15A25547):

   ★ How to Be Alone, by Andrea Dorfman and poet/singer/songwriter, Tanya Davis.
   ★ Embrace Life, a commercial for wearing seat belts (!)
   ★ Free Hugs Campaign, the story of Juan Mann, whose sole mission was to reach out and hug a stranger.

✓ Hugging, stretching, hand-over-heart meditating.

✓ Affirmative words include love, compassion, joy, trust, empathy, balance and harmony. Themes to release include distrust, guilt, grief, regret, resentment and self-loathing.

✓ Goddesses such as Kwan Yin, Amaterasu, Hina, Tara, Hestia, Juno and Vesta represent the "Primordial Mother" archetype. They teach us how to rally our self-love and respect, and to mirror this energy back to others.

✓ Use the Goddess-ence 100% pure essential oil for the heart chakra to crack open any resistance to love. Sweet orange reduces anxiety, lemon gives clarity, geranium and chamomile balances mood swings, grapefruit white stimulates energy flows, and jasmine absolute is an aphrodisiac that brings optimism and balance.

Speak the Truth...

Weddings rival Christmas for family politics. We're no longer dealing with the tidy nuclear family model from a few decades ago. Nowadays it's also the in-laws, out-laws, steps, halves, the half-step-cousins-once-removed... The dynamics of modern families require greater diplomatic and communication skills than ever before.

There are four types of communication: informational, emotive, persuasive and social. It is important to understand the tone and manner required for each situation, and to be mindful of your speech, body language, facial expression and tone of voice to get your point across effectively.

To aid the clarity of the message, good articulation skills are paramount, using crisp consonants, well-paced delivery and excellent breathing techniques. Yes, even the simple act of breathing can boost your ability to articulate well. (Revisit the Self-Centring techniques if you've forgotten how to breathe!)

Being diplomatic requires patience and discretion. It is being smart with your words; using them wisely to convey truth without injury; and handling negotiations without causing emotional distress.

It is beautifully described by Buddha:

If it is not truthful and not helpful, don't say it.
If it is truthful and not helpful, don't say it.
If it is not truthful and helpful, don't say it.
If it is truthful and helpful, wait for the right time.

Diplomacy requires careful consideration to the power of your words, and to pause and weigh your words carefully before speaking. This was a handy skill learned through baptism-of-fire by one of my brides recently. When her in-laws-to-be responded to the wedding invitation with, "When are you booking our flights?" she knew she had to get some expectations very clear, very quickly.

After doing some exercises to open her throat chakra, she finessed the right wording for her response in her journal. She then practiced her response verbally to her reflection in the mirror. Rather than having a melt-down about what to say to her in-laws, she responded calmly and rationally: "I'm sorry that we are not in a position to pay for everyone's flights on this occasion. However, we can assist with accommodation and transport upon your arrival in Australia." Easy-peasy!

You can be heard by speaking with authenticity and diplomacy, and share your learnings with grace. You can:

- ✓ Seek and accept help;
- ✓ Ask for abundance;
- ✓ Make your point without aggression;
- ✓ Choose your words wisely to facilitate understanding;
- ✓ Share insights that are precise, astute and relevant;
- ✓ Understand that your expressions manifests in exactly the way you describe;
- ✓ Aid effective communication between the genders, the young and the old, the experienced and the novice;
- ✓ Revert to natural and gentle ways of healing rifts and treating injuries.

Ways to speak your truth...

- ✓ Keep a daily journal, documenting your highs and lows. On the left-page write about your down days; and on the right, about all the things you have to be grateful for.
- ✓ Create a mind-map or vision board using images that represent your heart's desires and hang it in your personal space to remind you daily of your potential. No-one will see this expression of your truth, so cut loose with adding images that will make you wildly happy.
- ✓ Physical activities include singing, toning, speaking, letter-writing, cord-cutting and journaling.
- ✓ Use words around self-expression, truth, diplomacy and being heard. Themes for release include denial, unfair compromise, conditioned silence, old habits and lies.
- ✓ Take on a goddess role model that represents the "Natural Healer" archetype. There are many goddesses who rule over the domain of self-expression, such as Athena, Fortuna, Rhiannon, Dana, Demeter, Iambe and Oshun. They teach us how to ask for what we need, foster healing, settle differences and bridge the divide between the genders, the generations and the ignorant.
- ✓ Use essential oils to reveal your truthful Self. The Goddess-ence 100% pure essential oil for the throat chakra uses vetiver as a deeply nourishing promoter of opportunities and possibilities, cedarwood to decongest the chakra, lemon and cajeput to bring clarity and vision, lavender to balance your new energy, and frankincense to rejuvenate intentions.

See Beauty...

You have the power to make the world outside your head more beautiful because of what goes on inside your head. That is, you can choose to see beauty, both physically and symbolically, simply by deciding to do so.

Choosing to see beauty helps you naturally release habits of self-criticism and toxicity. You cannot be toxic if you're appreciating beauty!

Likewise, you can't be confused, lost or bogged down in trivial matters – your en*light*ened brain registers only the beauty you are focussing on.

When you choose to see beauty you can clearly know what is right for you, and act in honour of your innate wisdom and intuition. You can:

- ✓ Readily and easily move on from petty issues;
- ✓ Be grateful for your blessings, in turn attracting more;
- ✓ See and explore alternative views (and viewpoints);
- ✓ Live in a state of clarity by releasing negative elements that no longer serve you;
- ✓ Simplify your life, both physically and mentally;
- ✓ Make decisions easily and stick with them;
- ✓ Have regular bursts of epiphany, relish symbolism, and be grateful for the many miracles that present themselves to you every day;
- ✓ Self-reflect and find solutions by remaining open to divine guidance.

These are helpful skill to have, for example, when the mother-in-law wants to "help" with the wedding planning. (Remember, this is an example – in my experience mothers-in-law are beautiful people! Lord knows, I hope to become one myself one day!)

Seeing her efforts as "beautiful" (rather than annoying) helps you become calmer about the whole situation.

So what if she double-booked the hairdresser or mixed up the flower orders? These problems are fixable. A soured relationship built on toxicity is not so easy.

Having an attitude of "beauty" lets your thoughts be those of compassion, generosity, grace, gratitude and calm. It also lets you be aware of the many small miracles that happen around you every day.

I think photographers are particularly cluey on seeing beauty. Russell Ord, a brilliant photographer I've worked with on several weddings, once brought a couple to our Margaret River property for a shoot. I was gob-smacked at the results.

The old dairy, rusting happily since the 1950s, became a stunning juxtapose to the pristine couple holding each other tenderly. The dead tree on the back block became a dramatic silhouette behind the couple kissing at sunset. And the paddock overgrown with wild oats became a romantic, whimsical setting for the couple gazing at the horizon and their future as husband and wife.

To practice seeing beauty, therefore, one way is to pull out your digital camera. Re-frame old items as new, trash as treasure, or overgrown as designer-whimsical.

Ways to see more beauty...

- ✓ Imagine a stop-sign any time you feel your head getting cluttered with noise, worry or second-guessing. A person whose third eye is open is able to make decisions with clarity and absolute trust in her own innate wisdom.
- ✓ Become aware of signs and omens that present themselves to you. If it suits you, be guided by their messages. Deep down you will know what these messages are, what they mean, and what you need to do next.
- ✓ Physical activities include studying, teaching, meditating, decision-making.
- ✓ Here is your chance to create an affirmation that will banish procrastination and self-doubt for good. Focus on bringing mental and intuitive clarity into your life and on the benefits you will receive in doing this.
- ✓ Take on a goddess role model that represents the "Sacred Sage" archetype. "To thine own self be true," says Shakespeare, as do the many goddesses who rule over the domain of self-reflection: Isis, Hathor, Baba Yaga, Cerridwen, Brigid, Inanna and Epona.
- ✓ Use essential oils to open your third-eye and promote your willingness to trust. The Goddess-ence 100% pure essential oil for the third-eye chakra uses cedarwood unblocks energy log-jams ready for rosemary (a brain stimulant that promotes clarity), calming lavender, frankincense and lemon (for rejuvenation), and basil to assist with decision making in your new space of vision and insight.

Understand Bliss...

Any new wife will tell you of the difficulty she had sleeping in the lead up to her big day. Endless checklists tend to run through the bride-to-be's head, as do seating plans, last-minute tasks, and minor adjustments to the day's agenda.

Being able to sleep soundly – without the "late for the Church" type dreams – is a quality housed in the crown chakra. The crown chakra is the energy centre of bliss, of being connected to your faith and of feeling peace within. Considering it's located at the top of the head, it is no wonder sleep eludes the bride who lets the endless checklist clog her thoughts!

When you know, understand and experience bliss you can open yourself to joy; revel in your divine purpose/work with gratitude, dignity and generosity. You can:

- ✓ See yourself as a minute organism in the ways of the world, both in the physical and non-physical planes, in the present and the future;
- ✓ Be a cosmic traveller, time expander and a sacred vessel for divine expression;
- ✓ Intuitively and effortlessly share your gifts of wisdom, understanding and spiritual knowledge;
- ✓ Know your calling and honour your destiny;
- ✓ Interpret messages from Mother Earth via symbols; and
- ✓ Understand and experiences bliss, even if for one moment each day.

Taking care of your "spirit body" is paramount for peace of mind, the foundation of bliss. This parable of *The Four Wives* may demonstrate the importance of taking care of more than just your physical body and material possessions...

There was a rich man who had four wives. He showed his fourth wife his love by adorning her with glamourous clothes and the finest of jewels. Nothing was too good for his fourth wife.

He was also very proud of his third wife and loved showing her off to his friends. He kept a close eye on her, however, as he was secretly afraid she would run away with another man.

His second wife was the man's confidante. She was patient, supportive and gave excellent advice.

His first wife, however, was neglected by comparison. Although she was very loyal and worked steadfastly behind the scenes to maintain the household, the man paid her little attention.

One day, the man fell gravely ill. On his death bed, he thought of his luxurious life and how lonely he'd be without at least one wife to keep him company in the after life.

So, he asked his fourth wife, "During our married life, I loved you the most and showed you the greatest care. Now that I'm dying, will you follow me and keep me company?" The wife declined saying it would not be possible – she had a hair appointment to go to.

He then asked his third wife, "I have loved you all our married life. Will you follow me to the afterlife and keep me company?" The wife declined saying she was looking forward to moving on and re-marrying in the future.

The man was devastated to hear this, but asked his second wife to follow him also. Like the two wives before her, she declined. "I can only take you to your grave," she replied.

Just as the man thought he would die of a broken heart then and there, a voice called out.

"I'll follow you no matter where you go. If I were stronger, I'd even carry you!"

The man looked up to see his first wife smiling at him. She looked scrappy and starved, but when he looked closer he could see her inner beauty shining through the tears in her eyes.

"I'm so sorry," he said to her, holding out her hand. "I should have taken better care of you while I could have! Then you would have been strong enough to carry my poor, sick body across the threshold to our new life in eternity."

Every man has four wives, and likewise, every woman has four husbands!

The fourth wife is our body. We groom our body daily, washing it, moisturising it, exercising it and dressing it. However at the end, the body cannot follow us to the next world. Its destiny is to return to ash.

The third wife is our possessions, wealth and status. All earthly belongings go to others upon our death.

The second wife is our family and friends. No matter how much they supported us during our lives, they cannot support us in the after life – the grave site is the closest they can get.

The first wife is our soul. Nurture her, invest in her, spend time with her and make her strong enough to not just keep you company, but to uplift you for ever more!

Ways to be more blissful…

✓ Attend church, circle or gatherings. Go on spiritual and nurturing retreats. Create space for your Self. Create more space for your sisters.

✓ Pray.

✓ Watch the sun rise, knowing that this brings with a day full of promise. Watch the sun set, knowing that this seals a day full of blessings.

✓ Physical activities include sleeping, star-gazing, moon-bathing and cosmic surfing (imagining you're riding the milky way on a broomstick or surfboard).

✓ What is your highest potential? Trust that what you ask for is exactly what the Universe is waiting to bring you! Spread your wings and create an affirmation that is as uplifting and bliss- packed as you can imagine. Release guilt, drudgery, misery and doom.

✓ Take on a goddess role model that represents the "High Priestess" archetype. They help you see yourself as a minute organism in the ways of the world, both in the physical and non-physical planes, in the present and the future. Explore the more magical, cosmic and crone goddesses: Nuit, Spider Woman, Circe, Hecate, IxChel, Yemaya, Bast.

✓ Use essential oils to help you board the express train to bliss. The Goddess-ence 100% pure essential oil for the crown chakra uses peppermint, clove leaf, sweet orange and cinnamon bark to achieve a euphoric state of enlightenment.

In Summary...

There is no occasion, sentiment or sacrament quite like marriage. At no other time in our lives do we make such a solemn and binding promise of commitment to another human being. Marriage is an allegiance between two people in love, and a pact between like-minded souls to become even better friends with the passing of each year.

But as with all friendships, there are times of "better and worse, richer and poorer, and sickness and health."

True friends weather the storms together. They listen, learn and laugh together. They trust each other with their inner most secrets and wishes. They respect and encourage each other's individuality. They prop their mate up when they're down. And, they always see the good in each other even when they're feeling bad.

In the words of Arthur Gordon: "Nothing is easier than saying words, and nothing is harder than living them day after day."

Being a goddess for life, however, will give you the inner strength and fortitude to live your promises day after day, for all of your tomorrows, and the tomorrows after that.

Remaining connected with your inner goddess will give you an infinite well of resources to draw upon – a sense of belonging, creativity, individuality, gratitude, truth, trust and a connection with the divine.

You will be able to stand in your power. You will know when to offer support, and when to ask for it. When to listen, and when to give advice. When to speak the truth, and what that truth is!

And when you are standing in your power – in all your authentic, beautiful glory – your soul mate will have no choice but to say, "I do." After all, who wouldn't want to be nourished by all these gifts you bring to the relationship?!

And now it is time for me to say: Enjoy your wedding day, dear bride!

This is the day you will stand by the side of your love and offer your lifelong promise of love, trust and faithfulness.

In return, you will be offered the same, and the both of you will embark on the biggest adventure of your lives: to live the rest of your days as husband and wife.

I wish you well on your journey together!

With love,

Anita

About the Author

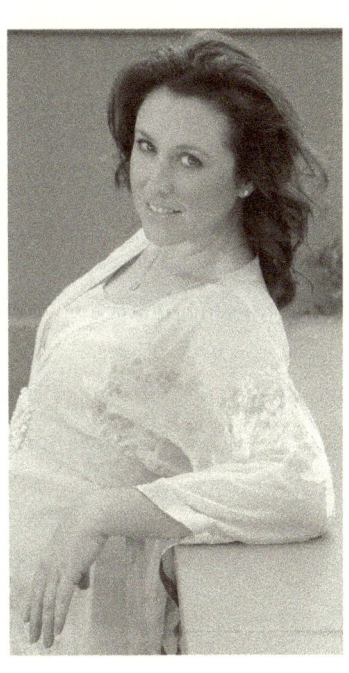

Anita is a creatrix, author, mother and wife, web diva, dream weaver, lover of life. She's also a Civil Marriage Celebrant, teacher, artist, traveller and joy junkie but couldn't make these rhyme.

These roles sum up her passion for inspired living. Her work helps you connect with your beautiful, sassy, intuitive, lovable, sacred and authentic Self – your inner goddess.

Anita lives on a farm in the stunning Margaret River region of Western Australia, but travels the world offering workshops and weddings.

Keep in touch with Anita via AnitaRevel.com

Other Books by Anita Revel

7 Day Chakra Workout

*What Would Goddess Do?
A Journal for Channelling Divine Guidance*

*BOTIBOTO: Beautiful On The Inside,
Beautiful On The Outside, An Empowerment Story
for Well-Rounded Women*

*The Goddess DIET, See a Goddess
in the Mirror in 21 Days*

The Goddess Guide to Chakra Vitality, 3rd edition

*Goddess Makeover, A Home-study Course
in Personal Values, Self-actualisation
and Divine Revellion*

*Marketing Made Easy for Celebrants,
Boost Your Bookings With Easy and Effective Marketing Methods*

Marketing For Authors

*7 Day Bootcamp for Brides
Feel Fit, Focused and Fabulous on Your Wedding Day!*

*Affirmation Goddess,
Express Your Way to Happiness*

And the number 1 free download...

The Inner Goddess Manifesto, 7 Rules for Knowing, Accepting and Loving Your Gorgeous Goddess Self

"The inner goddess is a woman's guiding light, her sense of self, and her moral and behavioural compass. She's the force who enables a woman to enjoy life as a confident, capable, sacred and savvy human being..."

The term "inner goddess" denotes the feminine aspect of a woman's psyche – her sense of the feminine divine and all the sacred and sassy aspects that come as a package deal.

In loving the inner goddess, we are allowed to be as vulnerable and soft, or strong and brave, as we are inclined to be. No-one judges us for our choices, because in being true to ourselves we inspire others with our honesty and light.

Reconnecting with the inner goddess gives us permission to receive as much love as we give and deserve. In being free to love unconditionally – both ourselves and others – we are allowing our inner goddess to flourish.

How does a woman reconnect with her inner goddess? One easy way is to acquaint yourself with The Goddess Rules and adopt them as your "rules of engagement" in everyday life.

The Inner Goddess Manifesto is available as a free download from iGoddess.com

---

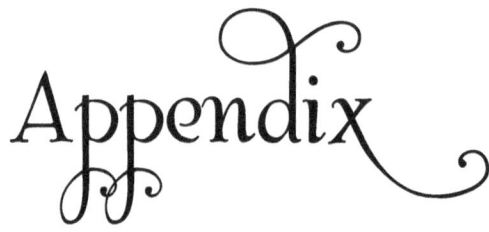

Appendix

Resources: Books, Articles, Social Media & Other Services

Resources

✓ The Australian government recommend 2.5 hours of moderate exercise a week. Download the guidelines: ausport.gov.au/fulltext/1999/feddep/physguide.pdf

✓ The United States Department of Agriculture has a comprehensive online database of nutrient profiles for 13,000 foods. You can find them under "Food and Nutrition" at usda.gov

Recommended Books

✓ *The Goddess DIET, See a Goddess in the Mirror in 21 Days*
~ Anita Revel (Now Age Publishing)

✓ *Goddess Makeover, a Home-Study Course in Personal Values, Self-Actualisation and Divine Revellion*
~ Anita Revel (Now Age Publishing)

✓ *The Goddess Guide to Chakra Vitality*
~ Anita Revel (Now Age Publishing

eBooks

- ✓ *Inner Goddess Manifesto*
  ~ Anita Revel (Now Age Publishing) from iGoddess.com
- ✓ *BOTIBOTO, Beautiful On The Inside Beautiful On The Outside, An Empowerment Story for Well-Rounded Women*
  ~ Anita Revel (Now Age Publishing) via iGoddess.com

Articles

- ✓ How to Write Your Wedding Vows. Read the article at yesidoweddings.com/how-to-write-your-own-vows
- ✓ Step-by-step guide: How to Get Married in Australia: GetMarriedInAustralia.com

Social Media

- ✓ Anita Revel on Twitter: @AnitaRevel
- ✓ Anita Revel on Facebook: facebook.com/AnitaRevel
- ✓ The Goddess DIET on Facebook: facebook.com/TheGoddessDiet

Services

- ✓ Find the perfect beach or forest and wedding professionals in Australia: GetMarriedInAustralia.com
- ✓ Anita Revel: Civil Marriage Celebrant / Officiant in Australia and USA: YesIDoWeddings.com
- ✓ Sandra O'Brien: Certified Personal Fitness Coach (Canada) muskokagoddess.com

www.ingramcontent.com/pod-product-compliance
Lightning Source LLC
Chambersburg PA
CBHW021020090426
42738CB00007B/837